Tactical Strongman

The Complete Guide

Josh Bryant and Adam benShea

Tactical Strongman: The Complete Guide

Table of Contents

INTRODUCTION

These days we prefer to train in the kind of isolated settings most commonly associated with the warrior monks of yesteryear or the iconic training montages of 1980s action films. However, sometimes, by happenstance or circumstance, we find ourselves in a commercial gym. Sounds, smells, and feelings invoke memories. It was true for Marcel Proust when he dipped a crumbling cookie into tea. It is true for us when we find ourselves surrounded by the clink of iron, inhaling the distinct odor of commercial cleaner, and touching the sharp edges of cracked vinyl on the workout bench. We are transported back to the old gym. To a time before social media dictated your workout wear, program, and attitude.

For those who read some of our earlier books, you have a sense of the way in which the gym served as more than just a place to move weight. It was a nexus of learning, a platform for success, and a portal for our rite of passage into the mythic world of strength.

Perhaps some of you had similar experiences with a gym from your youth. Such a place imparts a sense of fortitude that stays with you and aids you on the winding road of life. The strength you acquire from this place serves as a companion in your steady march of existence and keeps reminding you not to settle, to strive for excellence.

From our own old gym days, one lesson about strength stands out from the rest.

The workout on that particular day began in a most usual fashion, loading plates onto a bar and going through a mindful series of warm-up sets. In the midst of this meditative practice of strength gain, we heard loud banging from outside of the gym. Not ones to be deterred by noise, or any distraction, for that matter, we continued through our workout.

By the end of our training session, the noise had not diminished. If anything, it had increased in volume and frequency, and was now accompanied by what could be described as a series of guttural grunts.

Curious by nature and spurred on by the restless inquisitiveness of youth, we ventured to the outdoor deck of the gym. For those familiar with *The Saga of the Tijuana Barbell Club*, it was the same deck where later we would learn about interval training from Chato and his frenetic work on the heavy bag.

Farther back from the old punching bag, we saw on odd amalgam of stones, thick barbells, heavy plates, and a wide array of unorthodox instruments utilized for strength gain. Now, you have to remember this was before the widespread availability of internet search engines, and this predated the appearance of sleds and battle ropes adorning strip mall commercial gyms. So we were unsure what to make of the spread before us.

Moving our eyes from the training equipment, we saw a broad back adorned with a sweat-stained gray sweatshirt. A midnight dark ponytail rhythmically jumped against the back like the whip of a carriage driver against the hind of a horse. As he turned to lift one of the large stones, we saw his profile.

It was "Thic Vic"!

A legend in our town, Vic was a star linebacker and champion wrestler at the local high school.

After his senior year wrestling season, Vic cut out. He left town without graduating, and the legends about him started. It was said he joined the Army and got involved with all kinds of special ops–type stuff. We heard that he was on the ground during the infamous Black Hawk Down incident in Mogadishu and that he witnessed unspeakable atrocities during the Yugoslav Wars.

Thic Vic had shown up back in town about a year ago, and the mythic stories about him had multiplied. People said that he was making his money by taking illegal cage fights down in Old Mexico, where he used his immense strength and refined grappling skills to climb the ranks of the underground fighting world.

Before the term existed, Thic Vic personified the tactical athlete.

With the realization that we were witnessing a man of epic notoriety, we watched his workout with rapt attention.

Undeterred by us as his audience, Thic Vic continued to move through the workout with a feral type of intensity. Sure, we had seen the World's Strongest Man competitions on TV. But, in person, we had never seen anything like this.

Some key features of his workout were apparent. First, it was evident that Vic had established a predetermined order to his workout. Second, different body parts were worked in a sequence.

Third, while he would rest after he completed the entire order of exercises, he would take no rest before that. It was obvious that his symmetrical and muscular physique was functionally conditioned.

Viewing this spectacle of tactical strength became the catalyst for us to look into an unconventional approach to lifting, which has become known as strongman training. To learn more, we researched the history of strength training, and we refined the best way to train in the strongman style.

Here is what we discovered and developed.

A BRIEF HISTORY OF STRENGTH TRAINING AND STRONGMAN

The pursuit of strength has a long and rich history. In fact, some of the earliest recorded drawings of physical training can be found as far back as 4,500 years ago in Egypt.

When it comes to tactical athletes in the ancient world, none are more legendary than the Spartans of Greece. Before their fabled showdown with the Persian army at the Battle of Thermopylae, it is recorded that the 300 Spartans spent the morning performing physical training in the form of calisthenics.

While feats of strength are documented as early as the nineteenth century BCE, archaeology provides evidence of stories confirming the practice of stone lifting in the classical period of Greece. For instance, excavations on the Greek island of Thera discovered a 481-kilogram (1,060-pound) stone, with the inscription "Eumastas, the son of Critobulus, lifted me from the ground."

During this time, Greek athletes made use of unique types of dumbbells called *halteres*. It seems that these were used to aid in the distance covered while performing a long jump. Most likely, these are the precursors to the modern dumbbell.

In the world of Ancient Greece, few athletes were as renowned as the great Milo of Croton. His story is told by the Greek philosopher Aristotle and the great historian Herodotus, among others.

Remembered in popular imagination, Milo is referenced in the works of Shakespeare, Alexander Dumas, and Emily Brontë.

A celebrated strongman, champion wrestler, and revered war hero, Milo won the Olympic wrestling title six times from 540 BCE to 520 BCE. He also won seven Pythian Games in wrestling. Between these and other Greek national games, Milo won a total of 32 wrestling competitions.

His feats extended beyond the Olympics. At one point, he saved the life of the great mathematician Pythagoras when a roof collapsed on the man.

On the battlefield, he led troops to victory against the neighboring Greek city-state of Sybaris.

The idea of progressive overload can be illustrated with the mythic Milo of Croton. Progressive overload can be defined as the gradual increase of stress placed on the body during training. This could be done with more weight, shorter breaks, or longer rounds. Milo followed a training regimen characterized by small incremental increases in training weights that added up over weeks, months, and years. The legend goes that as a boy, Milo would carry a calf. With each day, the calf grew a little, and as a consequence, the weight on young Milo's shoulder would gradually increase. Over a number of years, the small calf grew to a large cow. Milo's strength grew along with it. So, by the time Milo reached manhood, he could easily hoist a cow on his shoulders.

Milo didn't start by carrying a large cow; he worked his way up from a small calf. It does not matter where you start, it just matters that you start.

Wrestling, dumbbell training, strength feats, and calisthenics were part of a holistic Greek culture, with its emphasis on a complete mind, body, and spirit. The Romans took strength training in a more pragmatic direction by looking to create a direct transference to martial ability.

For example, in a manner similar to the sledgehammer commonly used in contemporary training methods, Roman soldiers built functional strength by chopping at wooden posts with weapons much heavier than those used in actual combat.

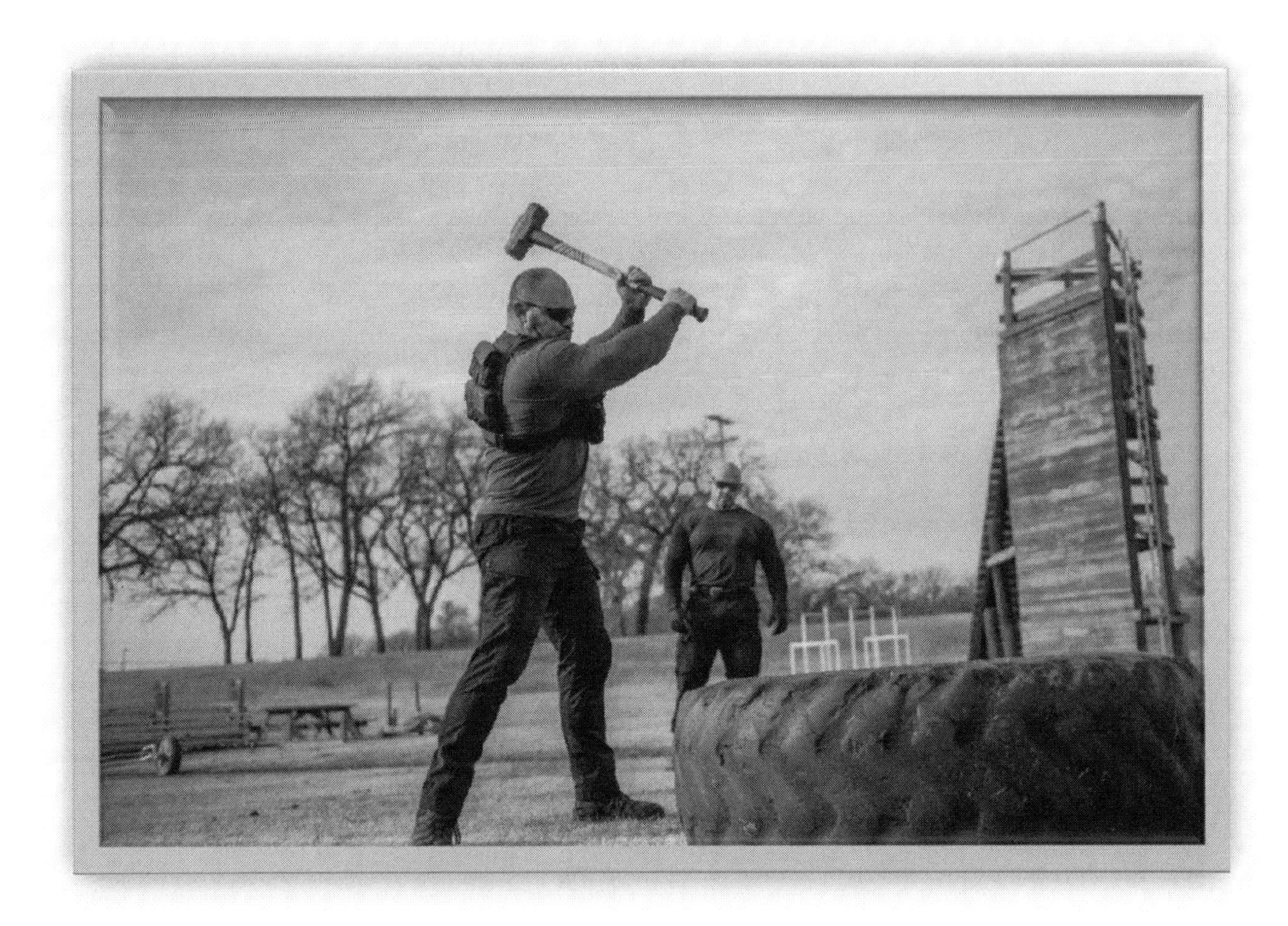

Butch Steinle Training with the Sledgehammer

A formal style of weight training began with the fearsome Roman army, and the programs they produced aided their capabilities as some of the earliest tactical athletes. Galen, a Greek physician living in the Roman Empire during the second century CE, cultivated a systematic approach to strength training. Using a system of heavy lifting and isometrics, he advocated a series of exercises to improve athletic performances.

However, a culture of athleticism and a methodical approach to the cultivation of strength deteriorated with the decline of the Roman Empire. Through the Dark Ages, physical training was synonymous with preparation for warfare. Every athlete was a tactical athlete.

Physical culture re-emerged during the Renaissance era of the fifteenth and sixteenth centuries, when boys were encouraged to engage in physical training by climbing ropes, lifting weights, and engaging in competitions of strength. Over the next couple of centuries, an interest in "manly" exercise increased in popularity and prominence.

After the first American gymnasium was opened in Northampton, Massachusetts, in 1824, weightlifting became increasingly common in the United States. Across the pond in Europe, lifting was even more popular, and we see a classic example of the tactical strongman.

Hailing from the region between modern-day Estonia and Latvia, George "The Russian Lion" Hackenschmidt is recognized as the first pro wrestling world heavyweight champion. He also invented the hack squat, introduced the bear hug, and popularized the bench press. He also served in the army as an elite guard of the Russian czar.

On May 4, 1905, Hackenschmidt became the first recognized World Heavyweight Wrestling Champion by defeating American Tom Jenkins in New York City's Madison Square Garden. He had immense strength, especially in an unorthodox type of lifting. For instance, from a wrestler's bridge, Hackenschmidt could grab a 335-pound barbell off the ground, bring it to his chest, and bench press it.

Well read, cultured, and able to speak seven languages fluently, Hackenschmidt was popular in social circles and authored several books. He was friends with the magician Harry Houdini and the Irish playwright George Bernard Shaw. Teddy Roosevelt, a proponent of physical culture, said, "If I wasn't president of the United States, I would like to be George Hackenschmidt."

Throughout his life, Hackenschmidt kept a strict diet and training program. He stayed away from cooked foods and maintained that "the purest natural food for human beings would, therefore, be fresh, uncooked food and nuts." He drank 11 pints of milk a day, while avoiding alcohol, tobacco, and coffee.

Hackenschmidt would rise at 7 a.m., take a cold bath, and dry off with a rough towel or with light exercises. From 8 to 11 a.m., he would have breakfast and take a long walk. From 11 a.m. to 12 p.m., he exercised vigorously. Lunch would be at 1:30 p.m., possibly followed by a nap.

He completed a second period of intense exercise from 5 to 6 p.m. and had dinner at 7:30 p.m.

By 11 p.m. he was in bed. On Sunday, he would not work out, but he would walk.

There are some important takeaways from his daily routine. First, he was disciplined about his sleep. Second, he maintained a regular routine. Remember, from our original bestseller *Jailhouse Strong*, these two of the Jailhouse Strong decrees: Get plenty of rest, and the body thrives on a routine. In addition, he stayed away from the jogging craze and other similar types of moderate cardio. Rather, he trained with intensity and completed active rest with his walking habit.

Perhaps the most recognizable strongman from this era, however, was Eugene Sandow. Known as the father of modern bodybuilding, Sandow created a popular display of muscle posing and strength feats.

Sandow's unique strength exhibition was discovered by Florenz Ziegfeld, of the famous theatrical revue Ziegfeld Follies, who brought Sandow to the 1893 World's Fair in Chicago.

Interestingly, Ziegfeld observed that audiences were more taken by Sandow flexing his muscles than the amount of weight he actually lifted. From this realization, the modern show of bodybuilding took shape.

In 1901, Sandow put together the first official bodybuilding competition. It was held at London's Royal Albert Hall, and the three judges for the bodybuilding event were the sculptor Sir Charles Lawes, Sir Arthur Conan Doyle (author of the Sherlock Holmes series), and Sandow.

To develop his own physique, Sandow studied classical Greek and Roman sculptures. He found a pattern of symmetry and proportion, which he referred to as the Grecian Ideal, and looked to develop his body in these exact proportions.

Sandow's legacy lives on in the world of physical culture. Most notably, since 1977, the winner of the Mr. Olympia bodybuilding contest receives a bronze statue known simply as the Sandow.

One of the greatest lessons we can take away from Sandow comes from the following quote: "You may go through the list of exercises with dumbbells a hundred times a day, but unless you fix your mind upon those muscles to which the work is applied, such exercise will bring but little, if any, benefit. If, upon the other hand, you concentrate your mind upon the muscles in use, then immediately development begins."

At Jailhouse Strong, we refer to this concept as muscle intentionality, or the process of bringing complete mental focus to your physical movements and the specific muscles you are targeting with a particular lift. From this practice, one learns consciousness-raising techniques that can be applied to any of life's activities.

Sandow impacted a young Bernarr Macfadden, who would later drive a physical fitness movement in America through his large media empire and his periodical, *Physical Culture*.

Contemporaneously, competitive lifting was becoming more popular. For instance, in 1896, the first modern Olympics featured weightlifting. Thereafter, in 1925, Alan Calvert (of the Milo Barbell Company) worked with Canadian strongman George Jowett, circus performer Ottley Coulter, and David Willoughby to create the American Continental Weightlifter's Association, which defined a full list of lifts, rules, and regulations.

Over the ensuing decades, two distinct lines of competitive lifting emerged. On one hand is Olympic weightlifting, which currently comprises the snatch and the clean and jerk. As the name implies, this type of lifting (with some variants) has been a feature of every modern Olympics.

On the other hand is powerlifting, which emerged in the 1950s and had its first sanctioned competition in 1964. This sport morphed out of practicing the "odd lifts," or the bench press, deadlift, and squat. Some of the early powerlifting pioneers were Bob Hoffman on the East Coast and Bill "Peanuts" West on the West Coast.

From the mid-twentieth century on, powerlifting and Olympic lifting developed into disparate strength sports. There were, however, the rare athletes who could make the crossover between the two disciplines. The great Paul Anderson made that crossover better than any other strength athlete.

Born on October 17, 1932, in Toccoa, Georgia, Anderson is nothing short of a lifting legend. An Olympic gold medalist, world champion, and two-time national champion, Anderson also had an integral role in the development of the competitive sport of powerlifting.

Paul was a teenager when he started weight training, with the goal of getting bigger and stronger for his high school football team. To build functional size and strength for his position as a blocking back, Anderson lifted homemade weights his father created by pouring concrete into a wooden form.

In a pattern seen time and again among physical cultural greats, Paul found a mentor.

Specifically, shortly after high school, Anderson met Bob Peoples, who influenced his squat training and offered an introduction into the broader world of lifting.

After winning the national AAU title in 1955, Paul travelled to the Soviet Union to compete during the rising tensions of the Cold War. When Paul came up to the platform where a bar loaded with 402.5 pounds was placed before him, the Russians snickered in disbelief. However, when Paul hoisted the weight in a two-hand press, the Soviet announcer's stoic manner betrayed a clear sense of awe as he reported: "We rarely have such weights lifted." In the midst of ideological, political, and athletic conflict with Russia, Paul Anderson stood as a powerful symbol of strength.

En route to winning the world championships in 1955, Anderson set world records with a press of 407.7 pounds and a total of 1,129.5 pounds. When Anderson returned stateside, then Vice President Richard Nixon thanked him for being an ambassador of goodwill.

Paul's winning ways continued the following year when he took gold in the 1956 Olympics (a feat he accomplished with a 104-degree temperature). After the Olympics, Anderson started earning money with his feats of strength. While he did display legendary levels of strength, the payments he received disqualified him from competing in the 1960 Olympics.

Nonetheless, he showcased his immense strength with unorthodox lifts such as his *Guinness Book of World Records* backlift of 6,270 pounds. His best Olympic lifts in competition are as follows: clean and press of 408.5 pounds, a snatch of 335 pounds, and a clean and jerk of 440 pounds. In powerlifting exhibitions or in training, Anderson said his best lifts in powerlifting were a raw squat off 1,200 pounds, a raw bench press of 628 pounds, and a raw deadlift of 820 pounds. Some of the other lifts he claimed to complete include a front squat of 930 pounds, a push press of 560 pounds, and a military press of 435 pounds.

Anderson is that rare specimen who was able to excel in powerlifting, Olympic lifting, and in what could be called "strongman."

Separate from Olympic weightlifting and powerlifting, it could be said that strongman is both older and newer than those types of competitive lifting. Unquestionably, strongman has a connection back to the earliest knuckle dragger who saw a big stone and felt an urge to lift it.

More recently, competitive contests of strongmen events began with the first "World's Strongest Man" in 1977.

The event was organized by two Scots, David P. Webster and Douglas Edmunds, who used their respective experience in the Highland Games and throwing to plan the competition. Held at Universal Studios in California, the inaugural show boasted a cast of bulky competitors whose skill sets are emblematic of the eclectic nature of the sport. The contestants and their respective disciplines were as follows: Jon Cole (powerlifter), Franco Columbu (bodybuilder), Mike Dayton (stuntman/bodybuilder/martial artist), Lou Ferrigno (bodybuilder), George Frenn (hammer thrower), Ken Patera (pro wrestler/Olympic lifter), Bruce Wilhelm (Olympic lifter), and Bob Young (football player).

To match this diverse group, the original events were wide ranging and unorthodox. They included the barrel lift, bar bend, wrist roll, tire toss, tram pull, car deadlift, girl squat, refrigerator race, and tug-of-war.

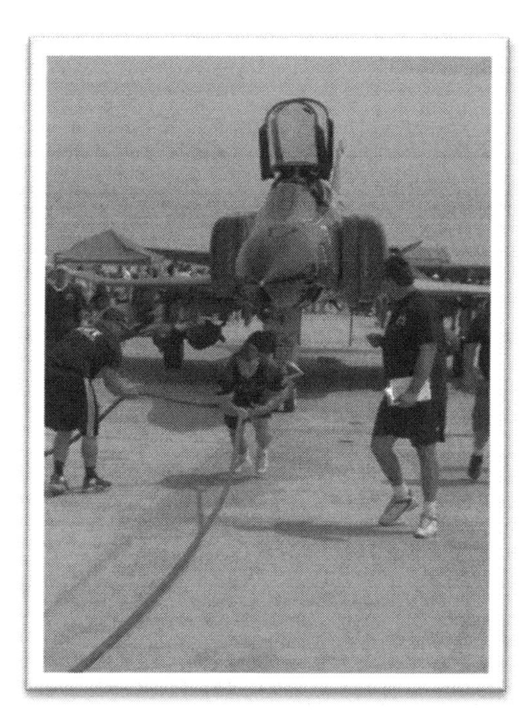

Author Josh Bryant Airplane Pull – 2004

In the end, Olympic lifter Bruce Wilhelm won the title of World's Strongest Man, and a wide audience was left in amazement, but also scratching their heads in confusion about how to categorize this new sport. Since that first spectacle of strength, the astonishment of the viewers has by no means wavered. However, there is now a systematic way to organize the strongman events.

To offer an approachable entryway of understanding for this growing sport and method of training, strongman can be characterized by six types of strongman events. In a general sense the events are divided among squatting, deadlifting, clean and press, loading, carrying, and flipping/pulling.

Examples of squatting could be fat bar squats or squats for reps.

Forms of the deadlift that appear in strongman include deficit deadlifts, car deadlifts, and deadlift for maximum weight.

Variations of the clean and press in strongman are seen with the log lift and circus dumbbell and axle for reps.

Loading is very common in strongman. Some examples of this include loading stones, sandbags, and kegs.

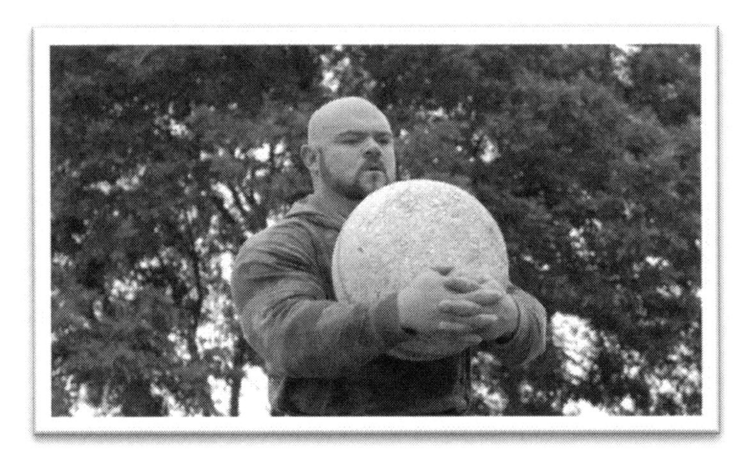

Butch Steinle Stone Lifting

The carrying element of strongman may be the quintessence of the sport. Some variations are the yoke carry, farmer's walk, and duck walk.

Some may assert that it is a little tricky to include flipping and pulling under one category.

However, both activities consist of moving weight over a distance without any type of carry.

This makes the two related to one another. An example of flipping can be seen with tire flips, and a common pulling movement is the truck pull.

Given the extensive array of strongman movements, it should be evident that this type of training has broad applicability and offers a functional mode of movement for a wide range of athletes.

Now that you have a general overview of strength training and the disciplines of bodybuilding, powerlifting, Olympic lifting, and strongman training, let's talk about the why of strongman.

WHY STRONGMAN TRAINING?

We watched Thic Vic's workout with patience and studied interest until it came to its end with the last stone being placed with a resounding thud. With that, Vic stood arms akimbo on his hips, overlooking the sweaty, chalked remnants of his grueling session. He seemed to give a slight nod in satisfaction before turning to us, his audience.

His eyes squinted in an attempt at recognition as he lifted his scar-marked chin inquisitively.

Over the past few months, we had been introduced to Vic and exchanged a few words.

"You boys watching me train?" His words came out like gravel dropping on cement, rough and ragged.

"Yeah, we didn't mean to interrupt." We spoke with respect but with more than a little of the hesitant confidence of youth.

"It wasn't an interruption," he said, shrugging off our comment. "You see," his palms were open and facing each other, as if he were explaining something complex in very simple terms, "when I train, I enter into a meditative trance."

"What do you mean?" Even as teenagers, we knew enough about Eastern schools of philosophy and religion to be familiar with the concept of meditation. But this seemed to be different.

"Well," he stopped before continuing, like he was searching for the right words, "meditation in any form is an attempt to find a sense of connective peace between self and the surrounding world. But I could never go for the sedentary practice so common among ascetics and monks."

This was the most that we had heard Vic speak. His words came out in a staccato of wisdom.

Noticing that he had our attention, Vic continued. "You see, I'm a man of action. My meditative practice needs to match my personality. This kind of training," he jerked his thumb over his shoulder as a gesture to the pile of strength tools he had just utilized, "is the only way I have found to achieve a degree of meditative tranquility."

"So, you train for inner peace?" we asked with more than a little incredulity.

Thic Vic chuckled slightly, which sounded like he was gargling with rocks.

"That's part of it," he admitted. "But it really comes down to the fact that I need my training to fit my lifestyle. Look, I'm not sure what you guys know about me. I know some stories are going around town. Let's put it this way, I saw some things overseas, and these workouts kept me safe and sane. Since I got home, I've been taking some fights. Underground stuff. Most of the fights go quick and hard. I need my training to match that type of violent output."

"That makes sense. What do you call this type of training?"

"Tactical Strongman Training." He spoke those words like he was sharing an intimate secret.

"Great name. So, it provides you with emotional balance *and* functional conditioning?"

"Uh, more than that," he said as he crossed his arms over a massive chest and bulging biceps pressed against his thermal workout shirt. "You know how it is. I'm not in a place where I can really settle down. I mean, underground cage fighters can't afford to be too domestic. You have to be feral, wild. That means I'm playing the single scene, and, no matter what anyone tells you, a hard, muscular body will always attract the ladies.

"So, guys, this simple method of training will get your mind right while also providing functional conditioning and giving you a physique that dominates the attention on the beach and at the pool."

The Why of Strongman

As our mentor and dear friend, the late Dr. Fred Hatfield, used to say about training, "There is good, better, and best. And strongman training is the best."

Powerlifting is limit strength, or how much weight you can lift in one all-out effort regardless of time. Limit strength is also your foundation for speed, agility, athletic endeavors, and muscular development.

Olympic lifting is explosive strength, meaning strength executed with speed.

Bodybuilding is maximizing muscle hypertrophy within aesthetic guidelines.

Strongman is the synergistic hybrid of all three disciplines.

As a training method or as a competitive sport, strongman demands and builds limit strength, mobility, core strength, powerful triple extension, grip strength, explosive strength, stability, multi-planar strength, muscle hypertrophy, and a strong posterior chain. Beyond that, strongman offers time efficiency, functional strength, body composition and conditioning, grip strength, explosive strength, and a really enjoyable mode of training.

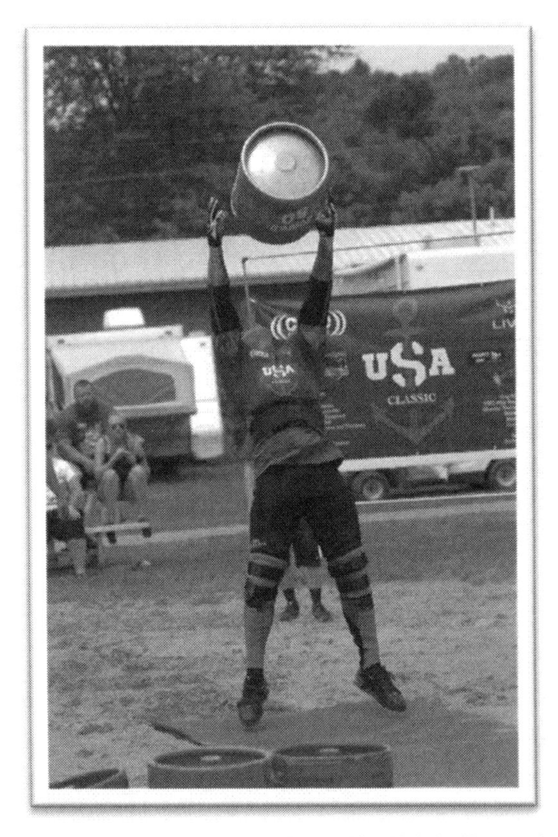

Matt Mills Keg Throw with Beautiful Triple Extension

Time Efficiency

Part of the beauty of strongman training is its simplicity.

In contrast, Olympic lifting is a little more complex. If you're fortunate enough to come across some old Soviet defector who earned the merited Master of Sport title, it would still require many dreary years under his Communist methods of instruction to get you to a level of competency in Olympic lifts.

On one hand, even under the supervision of a highly qualified Soviet defector coach, it takes a long time to acquire mediocre technique in Olympic lifting. On the other hand, strongman training has a very slight learning curve.

The wildland firefighter, infantry soldier, tactical athlete, obstacle racer, or just about any weekend warrior does not have the time to learn a sport such as Olympic lifting that is often more technical than their primary occupational or athletic demands. Further, even if an athlete is willing and able to commit the requisite time to learn Olympic lifts, this time could be more efficiently used gaining proficiency in their primary athletic vocation.

Think about it this way: Even in top-tier division one football programs, the best athletes in the country execute Olympic lifts with abysmal technique. However, there are junior varsity athletes "riding the pine" who can learn efficient strongman technique in one session.

Functional Strength

As seen on social media and the occasional "fitness special" on your local morning news, popular functional training is often a bizarre amalgam of "Sweatin' to the Oldies," Bosu balls, and pink dumbbells. The issue with many of these types of functional training is that they will not improve your strength, because you are handling light weight. To build on this, scientific studies show that training with less than 60 percent of a trained athlete's one-repetition max (1RM) does little to develop their strength.

Unlike other modes of functional training, with strongman training you do not have to sacrifice heavy weight.

Now, if you're an alpine skier, you may routinely require force production in an unstable Bosu-like environment. However, the same cannot be said for tactical athletes, the neighborhood bouncer, or defensive linemen. Therefore, it's time to pop that damn Bosu ball, grab something heavy and awkward, and discover what "functional training" really is—strongman training!

Strongman training helps you build strength in muscles and positions usually untouched in traditional lifting programs because it revolves around moving irregular objects. Developing those overlooked muscles, including stabilizer muscles, helps in your day-to-day movement, your other modes of training, and even when you are four sake bombs deep at the Don Ho cover band show and the Big Kahuna wants to do the toe-to-toe mambo.

Unlike machines or even barbells and dumbbells, strongman training requires you to lift heavy, asymmetrical loads in a multi-planar environment. You are forced to make adjustments in your positioning. This induces significant muscle tension in positions your body is not accustomed to feeling or exerting tension.

With barbells and dumbbells, the objective is to build a repeatable pattern because you are pushing, pulling, and gripping in linear fashion. This is not the case in strongman. For example, think of lifting a sandbag. The weight shifts in an unpredictable manner, just like a suspect being wrangled to the ground by an officer. Keeping with the sandbag example, your core and entire body work double time to stabilize the weight. Additionally, your grip is screaming as you hold and support the weight.

Strongman training can trick you into lifting more weight. In a 2009 study published in the *Journal of Strength and Conditioning Research*, the researchers found that during the yoke walk, strongman athletes showed hip abduction forces that were 112 percent higher than what they achieved in the test for maximal hip abduction. This happened because the force the athlete was producing by stiffening his torso to execute the carry allowed his hip to carry more weight than it normally could.

Training strongman events teaches your body how to fire its neurological system in a way that coordinates the entire body to perform supramaximal feats of strength. The type of strength that you build through strongman will not only help to up your powerlifting total, but it will also give you the type of raw power required to save a loved one during an adverse condition. You never know how the ability to move unorthodox blocks of weight will serve you.

Strongman training bridges the gap between the weight room and the field of play. You are able to build your posterior chain, static strength, dynamic strength, bear hug strength, and strength endurance in a multi-planar environment.

World-renowned performance enhancement specialist Joe DeFranco sums it up: "The beauty of strongman training is that there's no one way to perform the exercises. Athletes usually end up improvising to complete the event. The tire doesn't always flip over the same way. The sled doesn't always glide easily over the surface. The awkwardness of these events builds true 'functional' strength from head to toe. This enables the athlete to strengthen muscles that are nearly impossible to strengthen with traditional training."

Body Composition and Conditioning

Let's discuss how and why strongman training can improve both your body composition and conditioning.

Starting with body composition, how do you gain muscle?

Well, assuming that you are in a caloric surplus with a proper protein intake, most of your muscle gains are achieved by time under tension. Typically, in a program that is focused on muscle hypertrophy (that is, muscle growth), sets will take 20 to 70 seconds. It often takes a very similar time frame (20 to 70 seconds) to complete strongman events. However, in contrast to orthodox training with, say, barbells and dumbbells, in strongman events you are using much heavier weights!

Another way in which strongman training is distinct from more traditional types is the amount of time spent giving all-out effort. For example, in competitive powerlifting, you use your all-out effort to perform your one-repetition max. Of course, when going for your one-rep max, you will be handling a lot of weight, but you will not be in that crucial range of 20 to 70 seconds necessary for prime muscle growth.

In contrast, many strongman events are a test over time and distance. Therefore, in strongman events that are in the 20 – to 70-second range, you are handling a lot of weight and, at the same time, anaerobic lactic capacity is challenged. This type of training stimulates the highest amount of growth hormone production, which is a fundamental factor in building muscle.

It is mind blowing how much muscle you will put on when you repeatedly lift heavy loads in the 20 – to 70-second range. Moreover, you be working with loads that often exceed your one-repetition maximum in traditional lifts.

Strongman training is most effective for building the muscles that cap off a no-nonsense physique. That is, it builds slabs of muscles in your forearms, traps, and upper back. So strongman training gives you the type of build that can serve as a powerful deterrent, should you find yourself in a dark alley in Cairo's fish market or out for a nightcap in Ciudad Juarez.

These days, even the casual reader of supermarket muscle magazines knows about the effectiveness of anaerobic-style high-intensity interval training (HIIT) for fat loss. Low, slow cardio for fat loss has been relegated to the dust bins of history, where it is buried under high-cut Dolfin shorts and neon sweatbands.

Now, strongman training is traditional HIIT on steroids. Moving heavy weight in the 20 – to 70-second range, multiple times, is the most effective form of HIIT, and it beats the monotony of an hour on the Stairmaster.

Dr. Fred Hatfield said, "Life is anerobic." This sentiment is echoed in the research of world-renowned sports scientist William J. Kramer. In his research (found in the *Journal of Strength and Conditioning Research*) he stated, "Optimizing strength training for the warfighter is challenged by past training philosophies that no longer serve the modern warfighter facing the 'anaerobic battlefield.'"

When you are training for the rigors of battle, conflict, and intense athletics in any form, you must train accordingly. You cannot be locked into an antiquated and outdated mindset.

Professional MMA rounds are five minutes, professional boxing rounds are three minutes, and rounds in the fast and furious, now illegal in most states, Tough Man Contests are one minute in length. The average gas station defense situation is under 30 seconds; with the high adrenaline surge you will feel, it will come down to who can move the best without bringing in more oxygen.

Firefighters may need to carry a 300-pound person down two flights of stairs (mimicking the duration of a strongman event). Or a law enforcement officer chasing down a suspect and wrestling him to the ground will need to have an intense level of energy output for just inside of a minute.

Strongman training is one of the best ways to build real-world conditioning.

Grip Strength

You will never see a strong man or a strongman with small forearms.

While we've already discussed muscle hypertrophy, training for strongman also requires a significant amount of grip strength. This is because it is essential to be able to distribute a massive amount of force through your hands to complete many strongman movements. For example, picking up sandbags, farmer's walking with loads in the neighborhood of your one-repetition maximum deadlift, and performing various lifts and carries with abnormally large diameters to grip all require a huge amount of grip strength.

Improving your grip strength will benefit your performance in any physical challenge you encounter. Plus, increased grip strength has been linked with an increased life span and a higher cognitive function as you age.

Explosive Strength

The notion that the only way for athletes to build explosive triple extension strength (extension of the ankles, knees, and hips) is with Olympic lifts is antiquated at best and dangerous at worst! Olympic lifts benefit competitive Olympic lifters and elite athletes with personal coaches they work with on a daily basis. But, at the end of the day, for most athletes, the Olympic lifts are too technically demanding, are overrated for developing athletic power, and build little size or strength.

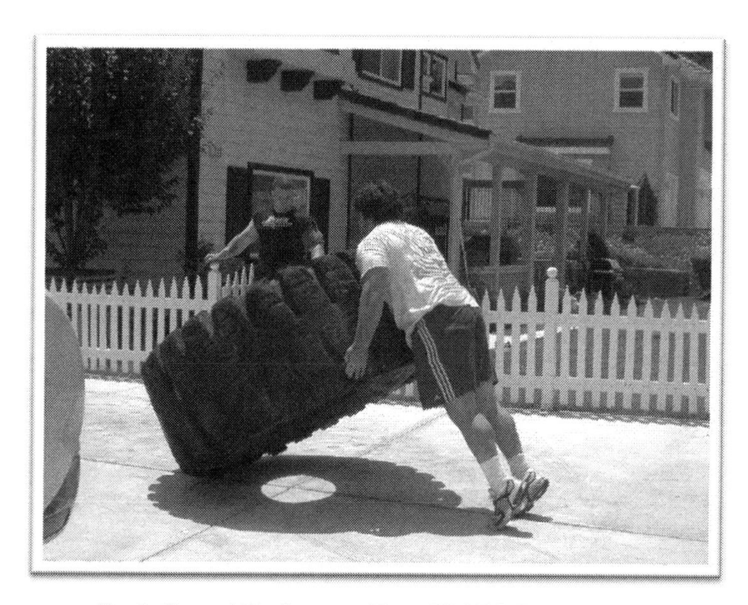

Noah Bryant Performs a Beautiful Triple Extension

Although there are some gung-ho Olympic lifting aficionados who are pushing their agendas to major certification bodies, coaches and athletes may benefit from broadening their horizons. In Plato's allegory of the cave, those inside the cave have a myopic view, seeing nothing outside of their immediate surroundings. Since the Olympic lifting agenda has been pushed for the last number of years, there are many strength coaches who see nothing else. However, to be your best, you cannot operate in "the cave" and simply accept the status quo. You must broaden your horizons. To get a wider perspective, we recognize that many studies show submaximal deadlifts (admittedly, not triple extension movements) to have similar outputs to cleans in trained Olympic lifters. Moreover, it has been demonstrated that trap bar deadlift jumps yield greater output than cleans in average athletes. Many strongman events require an explosive triple extension movement with odd-shaped objects in a multi-planar environment.

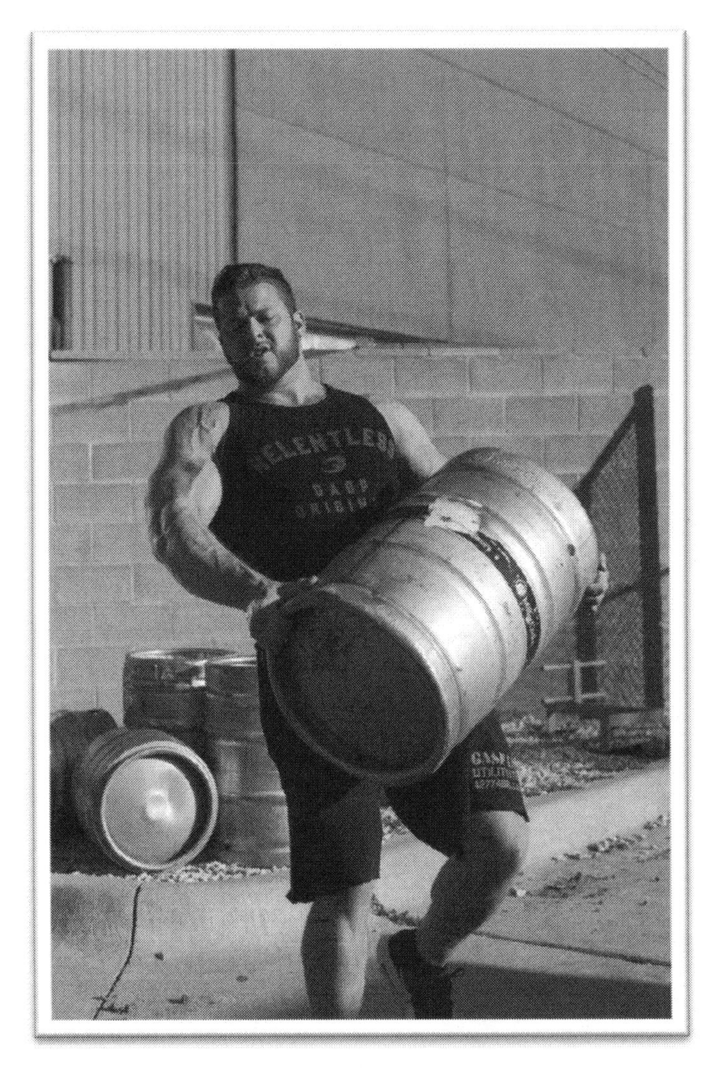

Austin Haye Lifting a Keg

Here are some strongman events that require triple extension:

- Keg Throws
- Keg Loads

- Throw Weight Over Bar
- Sand Bag Loads
- Tire Flips
- Atlas Stones Over Bar
- Atlas Stone Loading
- Tire Flips
- Real-World Tire Throw
- Any loading/throwing event

As Bob Jodoin, a strength coach and highly decorated ISSA trainer, says, "With stone lifting, you start with your knuckles on the ground and finish at triple extension. The loads and leverages are different, however, and this plays well into the concept of dynamic, real-world training. Good stone lifting emulates the perfect football tackle." Building on this, unlike an Olympic lift that requires a catch after the triple extension, after triple extension, loading requires that you push the object on top of a designated surface. In addition, a tire requires that you push a weight down after triple extension.

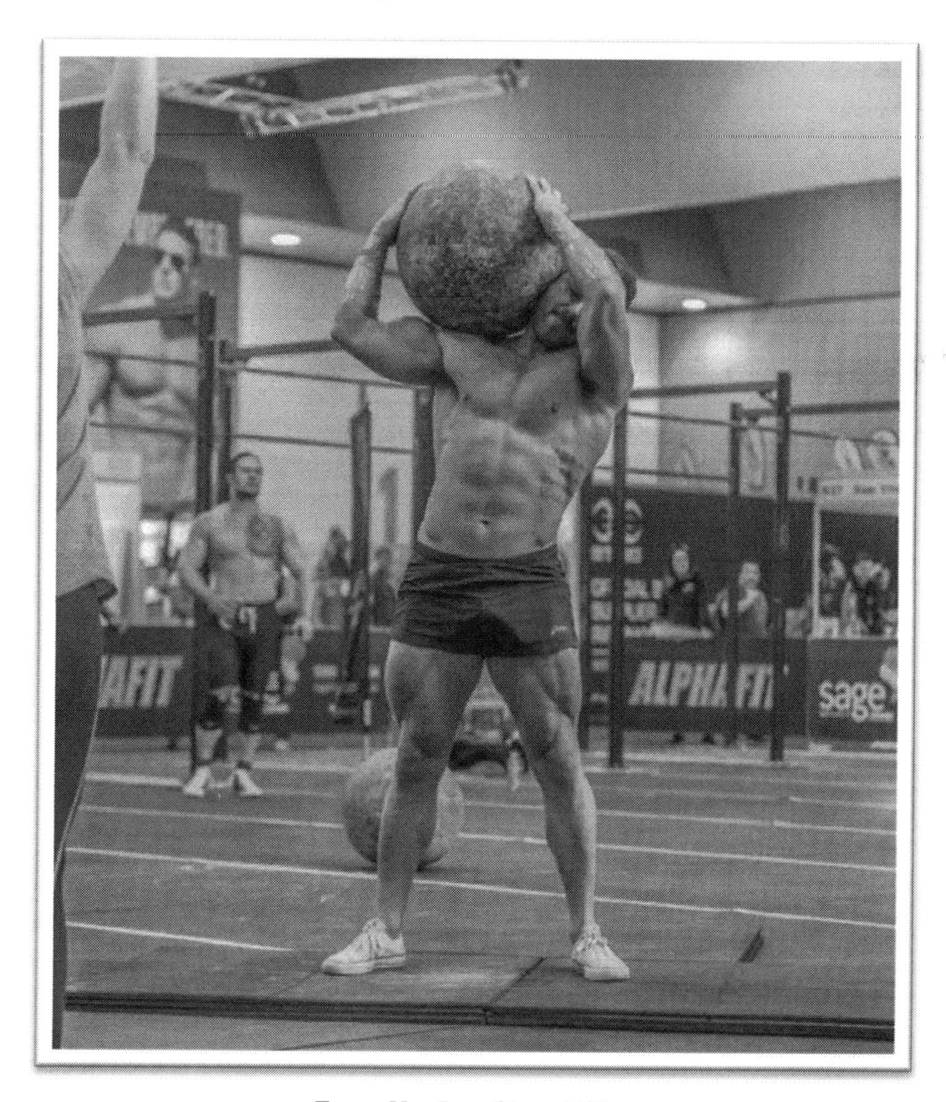

Tyson Morrissy Stone Lifting

When you encounter an opponent on the gridiron, in the cage, or outside some nightclub, will you drop to passive catch position or aggressively move through a triple extension with the type of ferocity cultivated by strongman training?

Enjoyment

The number one variable in deciding if a training program is going to produce effective results is adherence. If something is more enjoyable and mentally stimulating, you are more likely to adhere to the program.

When referring to strongman workouts he instituted at Michigan State, fabled collegiate strength coach Ken Mannie says, “It’s like game day every day we do it.” Bottom line: Strongman is fun and adds a new level of excitement to training.

The issue with “novelty” and “fun” is that they are often enjoyed at the expense of results. Yet, with strongman training, these work synergistically.

Final Thoughts

Strongman competitors are the strongest human beings on the planet. If they branched out from strongman for a prolonged period of time, world records would be demolished in squats, deadlifts, all grip events, and the overhead press.

In 2018, the average World’s Strongest Man competitor weighed 386 pounds, yet moved better than the average person who weighs 186 pounds. Programmed right, strongman events can aid you in any athletic endeavor.

It’s simple and brutal, and it can work with what you’re already doing. Or you can take the thinking out of the game and focus solely on your mindset by using our proven programs included in this book.

WARMING UP

General Warm-Up

If you are looking for an in-depth scientific analysis on why it's important to warm up, corner a doctor at your next cocktail party or plow through WebMD online. In the meantime, we will take you through a cursory look at the benefits of warming up and, more importantly, how to warm up.

Dynamic stretching will be the major piece of the warm-up pie. There are many successful athletes who jump immediately into our dynamic stretching routine by starting at half speed and gradually working up to full speed. We recommend that you start with a general warm-up before beginning a dynamic stretch.

The general warm-up is two to five minutes and should be something to elevate your body temperature. It could be an easy jog, a brisk walk, or your favorite cardio machine (if you train at a gym). Finally, after you complete the general warm-up, proceed to the dynamic stretching routine.

What about static stretching?

We recommend that you conduct all static stretching and proprioceptive neuromuscular facilitation (PNF) stretching routines *after* your workout, not before. Static stretching prior to workouts can take away from explosivity and strength. Of course, there are some folks who have performed these workouts with great success after beginning with static stretching.

Dynamic Stretching

Dynamic stretching incorporates active (meaning you actively stretch without outside assistance) range of motion (ROM). Dynamic stretches generally look somewhat like sport-specific or training-specific motions. Unlike static stretching, dynamic stretches are not held at the end of the range of motion.

A plethora of patterns can be utilized, but it's important to keep in mind that movements similar to those you will be training will provide you with the greatest benefit. Unless you enjoy being on the injured reserve list, here's another word of wisdom when stretching dynamically: Be careful to not exceed the currently established range of motion for the joint(s) being stretched.

There are two important details to remember to maximize benefit and minimize risk. First, establish an even, controlled rhythm, with all movements initially well within the current range of motion. Then gradually increase the amplitude of the movement until you are at the desired level of tension at the end point of the movement.

Remember, these are specialized movements, and care must be taken with their use. Make it a habit to precede dynamic stretching with a general warm-up of two to five minutes. To reiterate: We recommend not stretching a cold muscle!

Warm-Up

The following is an example of a warm-up for an intense workout.

- Warm-Up
- 2 to 5 min brisk walk warm-up
- Dynamic stretch
  - Walk on toes—2 sets of 15 yards
  - Walk on heels—2 sets of 15 yards
  - Arm swings—2 sets of 10 clockwise and counterclockwise
  - Arm hugs—2 sets of 10 reps
- Straight leg kicks—3 sets of 15 yards
- Leg swings—2 sets of 15 reps
- High knees—3 sets of 15 yards
- Walking lunges—3 sets of 15 yards
- Lateral lunges—2 sets of 10 reps (back and forth, do not hold end position)
- Wrist sways—3 sets, 15 each way
- Hula hip swings—2 sets of 10 clockwise and counterclockwise

Upon completing this warm-up, you start warming up for the first lifting movement of the day. To see examples of dynamic warm-ups, please turn to the Jailhouse Strong YouTube channel.

Some of the benefits of a proper warm-up:

IMPROVED PERFORMANCE!

- Increased muscle contraction and relaxation speed
- More "economical"/efficient movement patterns
- Reduced muscle stiffness
- Improved oxygen utilization
- Improved motor unit recruitment for all-out activity (i.e., more coordinated movements with increased intensity)
- Increased blood flow
- Heart rate is brought to the proper level for beginning exercise
- Increased mental focus for the task at hand, be it intervals or competition, by an increased "arousal," or enthusiasm, eagerness, and mental readiness

Warm-Up Weights

As you can see, the benefits of a proper warm-up are numerous. With a good warm-up, you can achieve more efficient movement patterns and increased mental readiness. Your muscles and joints also get primed. No successful lifter today forgoes this critical step. Why should you?

The warm-up moves in a funnel fashion from general to specific. After the general warm-up and dynamic stretching, you move to the specific phase. So, upon completion of the warm-up described above, if you're doing farmer's walk, continue your warm-up with farmer's walk. Use this same logic for log presses and dead-lifts—or any strongman event or traditional lift, for that matter. Warming up in a specific manner will get you mentally and physically ready to dominate the training session.

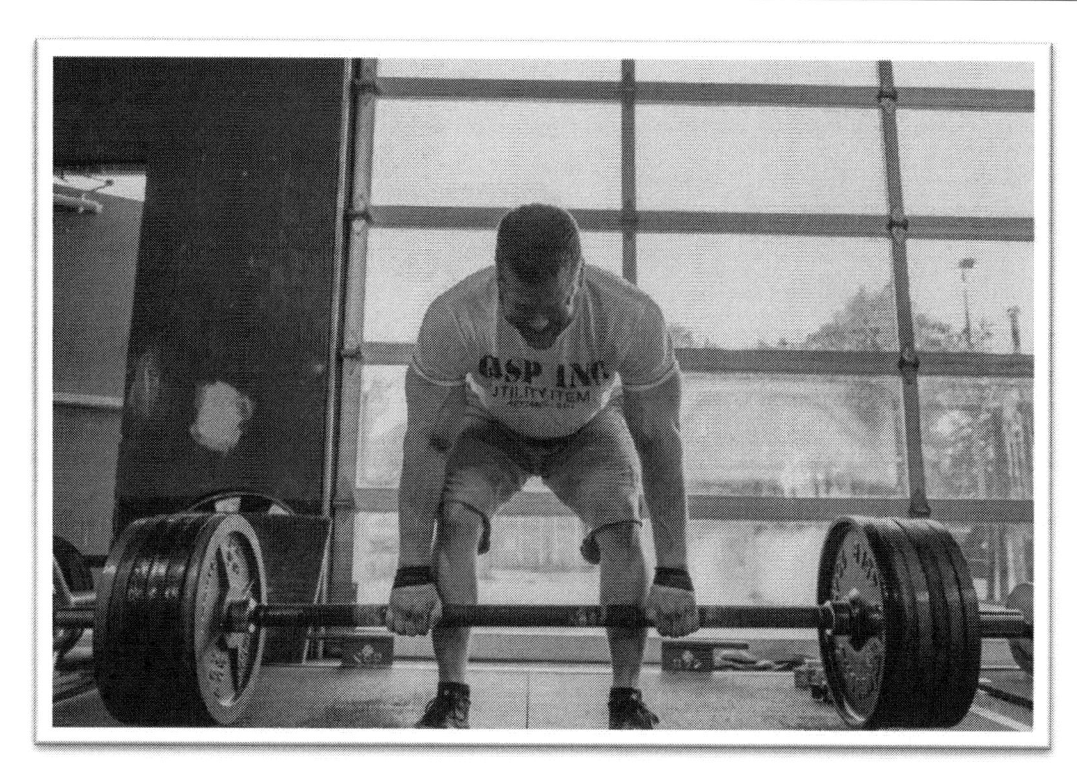

Austin Haye Axle Deadlift

An added benefit of doing warm-ups is additional volume. Volume equals weight x sets x reps, so loading stones with progressively heavier submaximal weights for 3 sets of 5 reps (where you are far from straining) adds extra training volume without adding extra time to your training session. Strength is a skill, and this skill is enhanced with a specific warm-up.

Example warm-ups for the first movement of the day:

Squats

45 x 6 x 4 sets
95 x 5 x 2 sets
135 x 4
165 x 3
195 x 2
225 x 1
255 (work set)

Farmer's Walk

75 x 100 feet x 2 sets
150 x 50 feet
200 x 50 feet
225 (work set)

Sand Bag Over Bar

50 x 6 x 3 sets
100 x 3 x 2 sets
150 x 3
200 (work set)

After you have warmed up and executed the work sets of a core movement or strongman event, you can generally cut your warm-ups down for additional strongman events to one or two sets (that set, or two, would serve more as a familiarization with the movement, rather than a need to warm up). We recommend one warm-up set with a submaximal weight for each accessory movement, just to familiarize yourself with the movement pattern you will be performing. There are more examples of warm-ups on the Jailhouse Strong YouTube Channel.

Final Thoughts on Warm-Up

Keep in mind that this warm-up is a good starting point, but you'll need to actively find what works best for you and what will get you warm for the activities at hand. While the need to warm up is validated by many scientific studies, the individual approach to the warm-up is an art. The longer you train and practice, the better artist you become.

BASE EVENTS

Programming, Training Effect, and Execution

All right, so you're starting to get the picture. Strongman movements are superior for developing functional strength, cardiovascular conditioning, speed, and sheer muscle mass.

Strongman training can benefit you in a myriad of ways. Functional strength can keep you safe when things go south during one-dollar kebab night at your local dive hookah bar. It can also give an aging Mr. Jones from Small Town Middle America the power base necessary to now carry home his bag of groceries (thank you, farmer's walk!). Or, hey, Candi the exotic performer can now lift heavy patrons up on stage for a celebratory birthday dance (thank you, sandbag cleans!).

Really, the possibilities are endless.

We are going to delve into four of the most common strongman events. Specifically, we will discuss the yoke, farmer's walk, atlas stone, and log clean and press. If you are able to become proficient at these four base events, you will become stronger, better conditioned, and hardened in body, mind, and spirit.

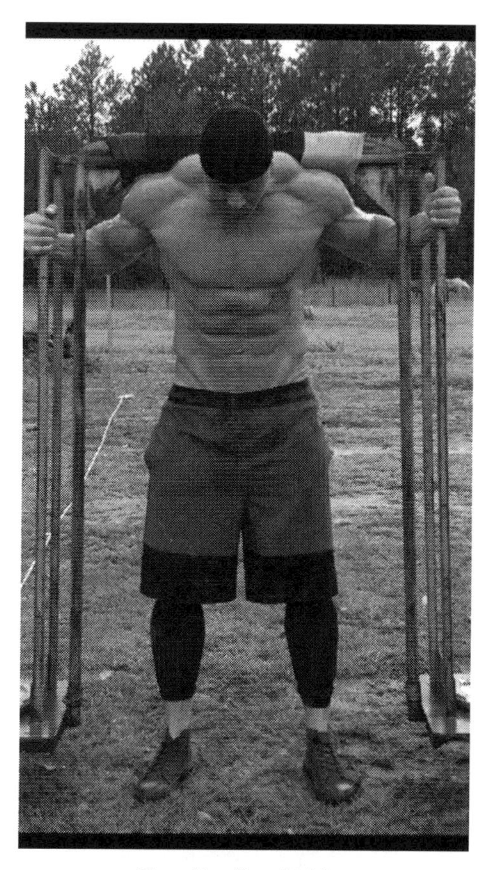

Tom Haviland Yoke

To get you proficient in these four events, let's discuss the proper execution of the movements, safety concerns, and how you can reach the intended training effect.

Safe Execution

Any time an activity goes from training to a competitive sport, the risk of injury becomes higher.

In fact, in comparison with many other types of competitive sport, the risk of injury is exponentially greater with competitive strongman. Even with light weight, a farmer's walk executed in training requires that you deliberately pick up a weight with good form, then you slowly begin the walk, and only gradually do you accelerate your pace. For an advanced athlete to win a contest, a light farmer's walk requires you to rip the implements off the floor and haul ass. This can throw off positioning and greatly increase the chance of a fall.

Now, remember, anything totally safe in competition is as useless as tits on a bull frog.

Nonetheless, we offer a list of six things you can do in strongman training to make it safer. In particular, non-competitors, take note.

- **Deadlift Double Overhand**. In strongman events, straps are allowed. So use them. Straps allow you to grip the bar with a double overhand grip without losing your grip or having to use a hook grip. With an over under grip, the most common serious injury is a biceps tear. Avoid this injury by going double overhead. You will also decrease your chances of other injuries and developing asymmetries.
- **Never Flip a Wet Tire.** Water on rubber makes the tire slippery. Not only can this increase the probability of a biceps tear, but the tire can fall on you or you can fall. In the same way someone trying to stay sober should keep away from honky-tonk bars, you should avoid wet tires.
- **Pay Attention to Friction**. Always pay attention to friction. This means that you should be aware of the surface on which you are training and the surface of the implements you are lifting. If a surface is slippery and it seems you may fall, walk away and live to fight another day. Or, if it is 95 percent humidity and 95 degrees outside and you are sweating like a woman of ill repute in a small-town church, avoid training with a wet, slippery plate or stone.
- **Technique over Speed**. There is a time and a place where a competitor needs to haul ass to win an event. But in training, the focus needs to be on precise, deliberate execution rather than mindlessly moving the implement from point A to point B as fast as possible. As technique improves, so will your speed. Remember what they say on the range: "Slow is smooth. Smooth is fast."
- **Technical Failure Is Failure**. When your technique breaks down, stop the set. In training, technical failure is failure. So stop. Going to failure and beyond may cause a level of fatigue from which it is difficult to recover. It also greatly increases the chance of injury.
- **Progress Slowly**. In powerlifting, it is unlikely for an athlete to go from a 400-pound to a 600-pound bench press in one session. With a yoke, it can happen much easier. Yet do not progress beyond 10 percent (which is a huge increase) each session, no matter how good you feel.

THE SEVEN GRANDDADDY LAWS OF TRAINING

There are some hard-and-fast laws of training that must be followed. These are not recommendations, they are *laws*. On the street, if you don't follow the law, you get thrown in jail. In the gym, if you don't follow these laws, there is a self-imprisonment of no gains! These laws were described by our mentor, Dr. Fred Hatfield, and must be applied to strongman training:

1. **The Law of Individual Differences**: We all have different abilities, bodies, and weaknesses, and we all respond differently (to a degree) to any given system of training. These differences should be taken into consideration when designing your training program. (This is why there are a wide variety of programs and variables presented to you in this book.)
2. **The Overcompensation Principle**: Mother Nature overcompensates for training stress by giving you bigger and stronger muscles. You can also acquire greater proficiency at the strongman events you are training.
3. **The Overload Principle**: To make Mother Nature overcompensate, you must stress your muscles beyond what they're already used to. Think about the famous story of Milo of Croton (described above).
4. **The SAID Principle**: This acronym stands for Specific Adaptation to Imposed Demands. Each organ and organelle responds to a different form of stress. Your body will specifically adapt to the strongman training demands you impose on it.
5. **The Use/Disuse Principle**: "Use it or lose it" means that your muscles hypertrophy with use and atrophy with disuse.
6. **The GAS Principle**: This acronym stands for General Adaptation Syndrome. This law states that there must be a period of low-intensity training or complete rest following periods of high-intensity training. Think deload/reload weeks.
7. **The Specificity Principle**: You'll get stronger at stones by doing stones (as opposed to, say, doing the yoke), and you'll get greater endurance for the marathon by running long distances (as opposed to, say, cycling long distances).

The more laws a program obeys, the more effective the program.

Strongman Reloads/Deloads

Why do you think most NFL teams have a light, noncontact practice before game day? It's to give their players a chance to rest their bodies—and their minds—before the big game!

Strongman is no different. You need to give your body time to recuperate after heavy training to prevent your joints, central nervous system (CNS), and muscles from becoming excessively fatigued and/or injured.

Reloading is the practice of following periods of high intensity and volume with periods of lower intensity and volume. It's also the perfect time to work on your form. We prefer the term *reload* to *deload* because it sounds more proactive—and because it ain't a blow-off week. Reloading is a strategic retreat so you can come back and attack some serious weight!

Reloads should normally be approximately 70 percent of the total volume and intensity of a heavier session. An easy way to make this adjustment is to cut all of your working sets down by one full set per exercise and multiply your working weights by 0.7. Voila, there's your reload.

Because you'll be using lighter weights, this is a chance to build your technique. It can be difficult to work on your technique when you're lifting more than 90 percent of your max in preparation for a contest. In reality, a reload week for the competitive strongman could also be called a technique reinforcement week.

Initially, we recommend reloading every three to six weeks, depending on how hard you train, any past injuries, and, of course, how quickly you recover. You can start by reloading every fourth week. Take note of how reloading affects your body and adjust your timing to meet your own needs.

As you advance, you can experiment with higher-intensity, lower-volume reloads, or the inverse.

This is about what works for you!

To recap, here's how to plan your own strongman reload:

- Reduce your volume (sets x reps x weight) by 60 to 70 percent of your normal workload
- Work on perfecting movement techniques
- Reload every 3 to 6 weeks. This is a guideline, not a rule.

Base Events

Let's offer a quick disclaimer: Reading this book or watching a YouTube video will never take the place of hands-on coaching from an experienced strongman or strongman coach. If you want to compete, we highly suggest you find an experienced hands-on coach. We wrote this to provide you with programming because, unfortunately, many who understand technique do not understand programming.

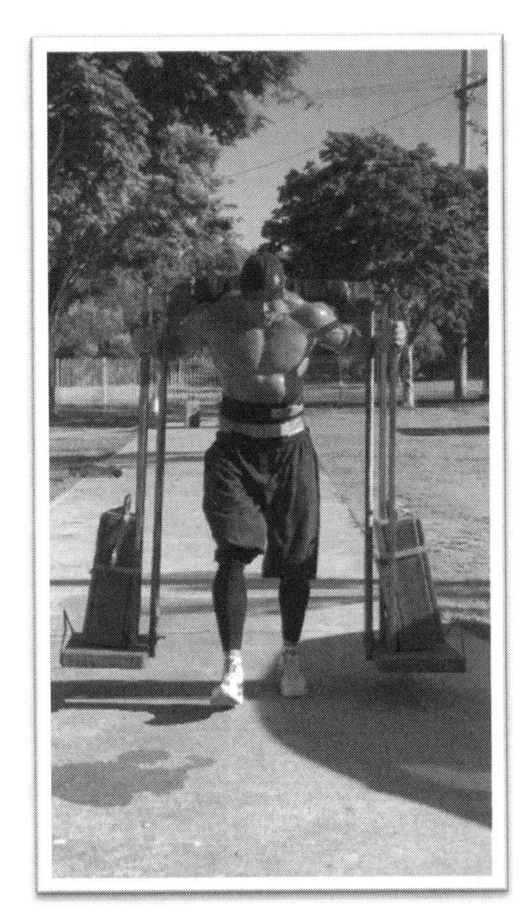

Tom Haviland Yoke

Yoke

A tough yoke walk can take more than 30 seconds. Often, the yoke weight is more than your true squat max. If you squat 500 pounds and have to do a yoke walk with 600 pounds, your body must dynamically stabilize 100 pounds over your squat max while you walk forward 50+ feet. In reality, you are overloading your system with more weight than you would normally put on your shoulders, while greatly increasing the time you are under tension. Your muscles will grow in size and strength, plain and simple. So the next time you try to squat 550, it won't feel so heavy!

In Competition

A yoke is carried for a preset distance, and whoever completes this distance in the fastest amount of time wins. When multiple competitors cannot finish the prescribed distance, the farthest distance gets the most points and from there points would trickle down in descending order.

Technique

Set up on the yoke crossbeams with a hip – to shoulder-width stance. When you stand up, there should be a clearance of two to three inches from the ground. After the yoke is picked up, you start walking forward. When placing the crossbeam across your upper back, pull your shoulders together (envision doing a cable lat pulldown with one cable in each hand). When you do this, a natural shelf is created across the shoulders and traps where the crossbeam can rest comfortably (remember, comfort is relative). This is the same position as a high bar squat. If it is too low or too high, it can be extremely awkward. There are three different hand placements on the yoke.

- Pushing out against the uprights from the inside
- Pulling in against the uprights from the outside
- Squat grip where your hands are placed on the crossbeam in a position that gets the upper back tight

Play around and find what position works best for you.

The yoke is a plank on steroids. Your back and core should be neutral, braced, and rigid. We advise using a belt with yoke loads greater than your squat max, so you have something to actively brace against. Again, when picking up the yoke, your feet should be in the hip – to shoulder-width neighborhood. Too wide of a stance or too long of a stride loads a single side disproportionately. This situation can make the yoke rock and become extremely difficult to control. From here, walk briskly in smooth, continuous steps. For the advanced competitor in a competitive setting, with a submaximal yoke to maximize time (albeit higher risk), you can start off with short, slower strides and gradually increase speed while simultaneously increasing stride length; this will not work with a maximal weight.

Training Recommendations

- For technical improvement—four to eight sets, 40 to 60 feet, with 50 to 70 percent of maximal load. Full recovery between sets.
- For maximal strength—two to four sets for as little as 10 feet, no more than 50 feet. Full recovery between sets; use 85 to 100 percent of maximal load.
- For hypertrophy—do three to six sets with 60 to 80 percent of maximal loads, for 50 to 100 feet (resting 90 seconds to three minutes between sets).
- For overload—pick up a load greater than 100 percent and do a static hold for 5 to 10 seconds, for one to two sets.
- In a traditional bodybuilding/powerbuilding split, the yoke would be performed on a legs or back day.

Beneficial Accessory Movements

The following is a list of beneficial yoke accessory movements: safety squats, Hatfield squats, front yokes, front squat static holds, weighted planks, squats, front squats, any specialty bar squats, unilateral farmer's walk, split squats, lunges wheel, suitcase deadlifts, landmine anti-rotationals, palloff press, barbell rows, and narrow-stance leg press.

The Yoke in a Program

Here is an example of the yoke integrated into a program:

Exercise	Sets	Reps/Distance	Rest Interval	Weight/Intensity
Safety Squats	6	3	120 sec	75%
Pause Front Squats	2	3	120 sec	65%
Yoke	4	50 feet	As needed	60%, 70%, 80%, 85%
Lunges	3	6	90 sec	Maximum
GHR	5	5	60 sec	Maximum
Ab Wheel	3	8	60 sec	Bodyweight

Farmer's Walk

Some variation of the farmer's walk can be found in the back alleys behind notorious Nordic Beer Halls, at the fabled "Basque Stomp," during the ammo can carry in the Marine's Combat Fitness Test at virtually every bush league strongman contest, and as a central component of the pinnacle strongman competition, The World's Strongest Man event.

The farmer's walk will help anything that requires explosive power, athleticism, grip strength, overall limit strength, and core strength. So, basically, the farmer's walk is the epitome of functional training for just about anything.

Many folks classify farmer's walks as a grip test. It's true that at the higher levels of strongman, grip strength may be the limiting factor for the well-proportioned, well-trained athlete. However, the farmer's walk builds the entire body. For instance, we have yet to meet someone great at the farmer's walk who did not have a big, beautifully developed set of traps. Furthermore, core stability, leg strength, calf strength, and the strength of the entire posterior chain (back side of the body) will be put to the test by the farmer's walk.

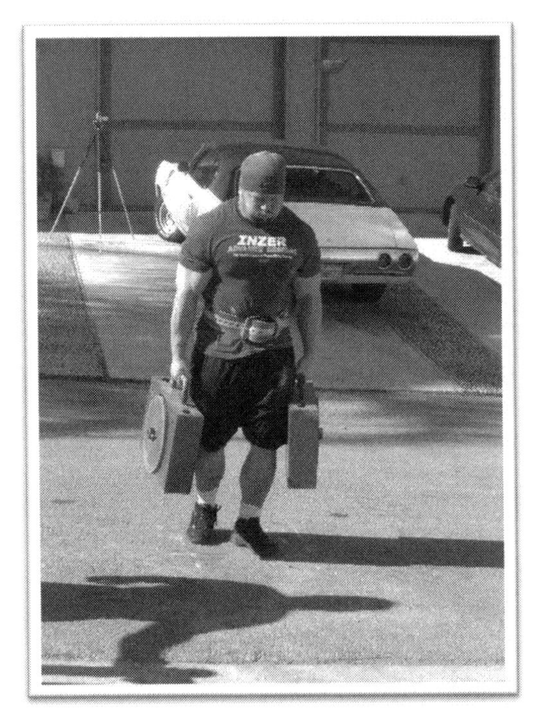

Author Josh Bryant Farmer's Walk – 2004

In Competition

In competition, the farmer's walk is conducted in a manner very similar to the yoke. Generally, it will be performed for a set distance, with the fastest time winning. If multiple athletes drop the farmer's walk implements before the finish line, placings will be established by the farthest distance travelled in a descending order. Sometimes, however, the contest will be the heaviest load carried for a preset distance (usually a short distance). At other times, the farthest distance with a preset weight will establish winners and placings. Farmer's walks, or a variation of them, are often a part of strongman medleys (two or more combined events).

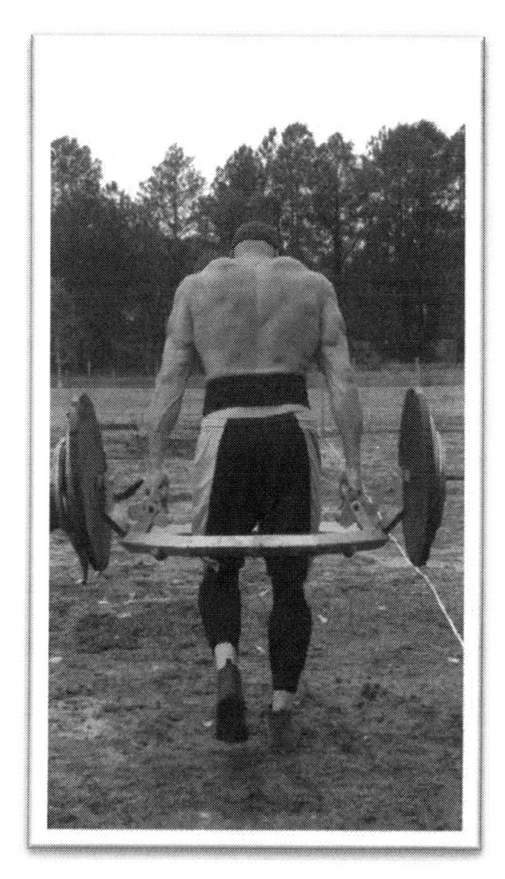

Tom Haviland Frame Carry

Technique

Set the handles so that you have a direct line from your shoulder to the handle, while giving yourself room to stand in the middle between the weights. Setting the handles too wide makes the weights difficult to pick up and unstable.

Remember to chalk your hands before picking up the handles. As you stand between the implements with your arms by your sides, depress your shoulders. DO NOT SHRUG UP! Brace your lats and core. From here, make your arms as long as possible while keeping your torso rigid.

Now, essentially do a trap bar deadlift from the ground while making sure that the handles sit tightly in the middle of your palms. With a tight grip, stand up.

Let the weight settle. Then move in small, even steps, making sure your feet remain beneath your hips; the more experienced you are, the faster these steps should be. By keeping rhythmically smooth steps, you'll keep the implements from bouncing around. If you are an advanced athlete using lighter weights, you can gradually increase your stride length.

Training Recommendations

- For technical improvement—4 to 10 sets, 40 to 60 feet, with 50 to 70 percent of maximal load. Full recovery between sets.
- For maximal strength—two to five sets for as little as 10 feet, no more than 50 feet. Full recovery between sets, use 85 to 100 percent of maximal load.
- For hypertrophy—do two to four sets with 65 to 85 percent of maximal loads, for 30 to 60 seconds straight (resting two seconds to three minutes between sets). Wear straps so grip does not limit you.
- For overload—pick up a load greater than 100 percent and do a static hold for 5 to 10 seconds, for one to two sets. If grip limits you, carry supramaximal loads with straps.
- In a traditional bodybuilding/powerbuilding split, the farmer's walk would be performed on a legs or back day.

Beneficial Accessory Movements

The following is a list of beneficial farmer's walk accessory movements: deadlift, overhand deadlift, trap bar deadlift, frame deadlift, finger plate pinches, unilateral farmer's walk, shrugs, frame carries, loaded wheelbarrow carries, and dead squats.

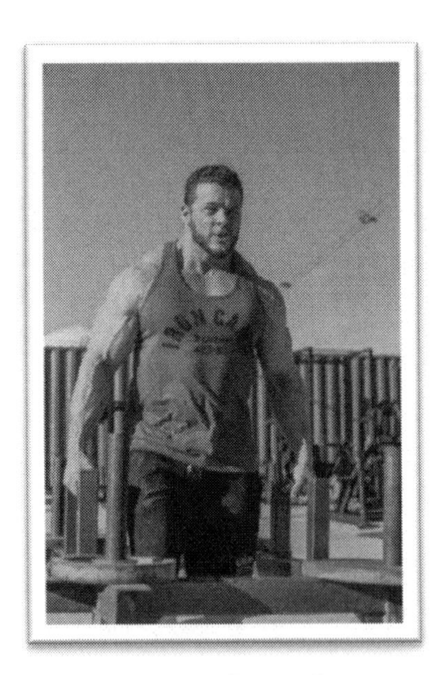

Austin Haye Frame Carry

The Farmer's Walk in a Program

Here is an example of the farmer's walk integrated into a program:

Day 1/Week 1

Exercise	Sets	Reps/Distance	Rest Interval	Weight/Intensity
Squats	1	3		85%
Speed Squats	4	3	120 sec	70%
Deadlifts	15	1	30 sec	65%
Pause Front Squats	3	3	150 sec	Max
GHR	3	5	60 sec	Max
Palloff Press	3	6	45 sec	Max

Day 1/Week 2

Exercise	Sets	Reps/Distance	Rest Interval	Weight/Intensity
Squats	1	3		87.5%
Speed Squats	5	3	120 sec	70%
Deadlifts	1	2		90%
Speed Deadlifts	6	2	90 sec	75%
Pause Front Squats	2	3	150 sec	Max
GHR	3	6	60 sec	Max
Palloff Press	3	6	45 sec	Max

Day 1/Week 3

Exercise	Sets	Reps/Distance	Rest Interval	Weight/Intensity
Squats	6	6	180 sec	75%
Deadlifts	15	1	30 sec	72.5%
Pause Front Squats	2	3	150 sec	Max
GHR	3	6	60 sec	Max
Palloff Press	3	6	45 sec	Max

Day 1/Week 4—Reload Following Prescribed Instructions

Day 1/Week 5

Exercise	Sets	Reps/Distance	Rest Interval	Weight/Intensity
Squats	1	2		90%
Speed Squats	5	3	120 sec	70%
Deadlifts Reverse Band	3	1	As needed/full recovery	Max out reverse band off the floor with 20% of 1 RM; i.e., a 500 max would be 100 pounds off the floor
Pause Zercher Squats	3	3	150 sec	Max
One-Leg RDL	3	3	60 sec	Max
Landmine Anti-Rotationals	3	6	45 sec	Max

Day 1/Week 6

Exercise	Sets	Reps/Distance	Rest Interval	Weight/Intensity
Squats	6	6	180 sec	77.5%
Deadlifts	15	1	30 sec	75%
Pause Zercher Squats	3	3	150 sec	Max
One-Leg RDL	3	3	60 sec	Max
Landmine Anti-Rotationals	3	6	45 sec	Max

Day 1/Week 7

Exercise	Sets	Reps/Distance	Rest Interval	Weight/Intensity
Squats	1	2		92.5%
Speed Squats	3	3	120 sec	75%
Deadlifts Against Chains	3	1	As needed/full recovery	Max out against chains with 15% of 1 RM; i.e., a 500 max would be 75 pounds of chain
Pause Zercher Squats	3	6	150 sec	Max
One-Leg RDL	3	3	60 sec	Max
Landmine Anti-Rotationals	3	6	45 sec	Max

Day 1/Week 8—Reload Following Prescribed Instructions

Days 2 and 5, Weeks 1-8

- Jump Rope—Four sets (20 seconds to one minute). Equal work-to-rest ratio, focus on fast feet
- Tempo Runs—Run 70 percent of max speed for 40 to 80 yards x 6 to 20 sets, rest 20 to 90 seconds between sets
- Dot Drills—Three sets of each of the following drills: up and back, right foot, left foot, both feet, turn around
- Pro Agility Drill—70 to 85 percent x three to six sets (rest 20 to 45 seconds)

As you progress, you can increase intensity and volume. This session is beyond active recovery, but not a balls-out session. It should take no more than 45 minutes. This type of work is a good addition to any program when you are bulking, while still maintaining speed and agility (which is crucial to strongman).

Day 3/Week 1

Exercise	Sets	Reps/Distance	Rest Interval	Weight/Intensity
Overhead Press	15	1 (last set max reps)	30 sec	70%
Pull-Ups	5	5	120 sec	Max
Dips	3	6	150 sec	Max
Overhead Dicks Press	3	12	120 sec	Max
Seal rows	4	8	90 sec	Max
Ez Curl 21s	3	7—7—7	60 sec	Max
Side Planks	3	15 sec	30 sec	BW

Day 3/Week 2

Exercise	Sets	Reps/Distance	Rest Interval	Weight/Intensity
Overhead Press	15	1 (last set max reps)	30 sec	75%
Pull-Ups	5	4	120 sec	Max
Dips	3	8	150 sec	Max
Overhead Dicks Press	3	12,10,8	120 sec	Max
Seal rows	4	6	90 sec	Max
Ez Curl 21s	3	7—7—7	60 sec	Max
Side Planks	3	15 sec	30 sec	BW

Day 3/Week 3

Exercise	Sets	Reps/Distance	Rest Interval	Weight/Intensity
Overhead Press	15	1 (last set max reps)	30 sec	80%
Pull-Ups	5	3	120 sec	Max
Dips	3	5	150 sec	Max
Overhead Dicks Press	3	10,8,6	120 sec	Max
Seal rows	4	5	90 sec	Max
Ez Curl 21s	3	7—7—7	60 sec	Max
Side Planks	3	15 sec	30 sec	BW

Day 3/Week 4—Reload Following Prescribed Instructions

Day 3/Week 5

Exercise	Sets	Reps/Distance	Rest Interval	Weight/Intensity
Overhead Press	10	1 (last set max reps)	40 sec	82.5%
Pull-Ups	5	4	120 sec	Max
Close-Grip Bench Press	3	5	150 sec	Max
Overhead Dicks Press	3	15	120 sec	Max
Seal rows	4	6	90 sec	Max
Incline Dumbbell Curls	3	12	60 sec	Max
Side Planks	3	15 sec	30 sec	BW

Day 3/Week 6

Exercise	Sets	Reps/Distance	Rest Interval	Weight/Intensity
Overhead Press	8	1 (last set max reps)	45 sec	85%
Pull-Ups	5	6	120 sec	Max
Close-Grip Bench Press	3	4	150 sec	Max
Overhead Dicks Press	3	12	120 sec	Max
Seal rows	4	8	90 sec	Max
Incline Dumbbell Curls	3	15	60 sec	Max
Side Planks	3	15 sec	30 sec	BW

Day 3/Week 7

Exercise	Sets	Reps/Distance	Rest Interval	Weight/Intensity
Overhead Press	6	1 (last set max reps)	60 sec	90%
Pull-Ups	2	6	120 sec	Max
Close-Grip Bench Press	3	6	150 sec	Max
Overhead Dicks Press	3	10	120 sec	Max
Seal rows	4	8	90 sec	Max
Incline Dumbbell Curls	3	12	60 sec	Max
Side Planks	3	15 sec	30 sec	BW

Day 3/Week 8—Reload Following Prescribed Instructions

Day 5/Week 1

Exercise	Sets	Reps/Distance	Rest Interval	Weight/Intensity
Farmer's Walk	4	50 feet	As needed	70,80,90.95%
Log Clean and Press	3	6	150 sec	70%
Sled Drags	6	50 feet	60 sec	70%
Stones	3	5	90 sec	65%
Juarez Valley 20 Squats	1	20—1	8-foot walk	BW

Day 5/Week 2

Exercise	Sets	Reps/Distance	Rest Interval	Weight/Intensity
Farmer's Walk	4	80 feet	120 sec	60%
Tire Flips	3	3	As needed	80,90,100%
Axle Clean and Press	3	3	As needed	Heavy as possible
Conan's Wheel	4	30 seconds straight	90 sec	65%
Triceps Ladder	1	100		BW

Day 5/Week 3

Exercise	Sets	Reps/Distance	Rest Interval	Weight/Intensity
Farmer's Walk	4	100 feet, 60 feet, 40 feet, 20 feet	120 sec	60%, 80%, 100%, heavy as possible with straps
Power Stairs	3	3	As needed	80,90,100%
Stones	3	3	As needed	Heavy as possible
Circus Dumbbell Clean and Press	3	8	90 sec	65%
Juarez Valley 15 Push-Ups	1	15—1	8 feet	BW

Day 5/Week 4—Reload Following Prescribed Instructions

Day 5/Week 5

Exercise	Sets	Reps/Distance	Rest Interval	Weight/Intensity
Farmer's Walk	4	120 feet	60 sec	50%
Yoke	4	100 feet, 60 feet, 40 feet, 20 feet	As needed	60%, 80%, 100%, heavy as possible
Axle Clean and Press	3	1	As needed	Heavy as possible
Viking Press	4	Max	30 sec	75%, 65%, 55%, 45%
Juarez Valley 20 Squats	1	20—1	8 feet	BW

Day 5/Week 6

Exercise	Sets	Reps/Distance	Rest Interval	Weight/Intensity
Farmer's Walk	3	50 feet	As needed	80%, 90%, attempt new max
Sandbag Carry/ Husafell Carry Medley	4	100 feet each	150 sec	70%
Log Clean and Press	3	1	As needed	Heavy as possible
Crucifix Hold	2	60 sec	120 sec	Heavy as possible
Biceps Ladder	1	100	None	BW

Day 5/Week 7

Exercise	Sets	Reps/Distance	Rest Interval	Weight/Intensity
Farmer's Walk	4	80 feet	120 sec	70%
Yoke	4	50 feet	120 sec	80%
Stones	3	10	As needed	Heavy as possible
Yoke Press	4	4	120 sec	Heavy as possible
Juarez Valley 20 Squats	1	20—1	8 feet	BW

Day 5/Week 8—Reload Following Prescribed Instructions

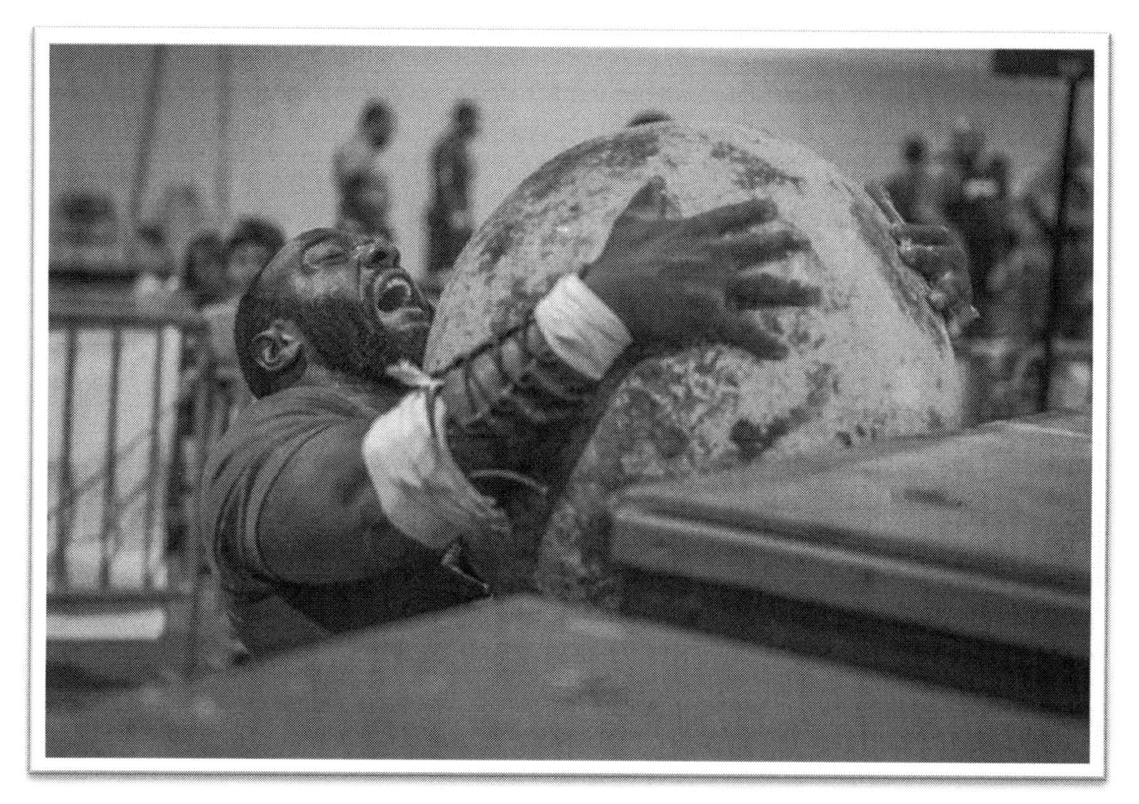

Mark Jones Atlas Stones

Atlas Stones

Picking up stones was a rite of passage for the Vikings. Stone-lifting variations have been popular throughout history in Icelandic and Scottish athletic events, and, of course, we cannot forget about the *Harris-jasotze*, or "Stone Lifters," in the mountainous Basque region, who gather in competitions held in town squares to find out who is the strongest! Atlas stones are spherical, like the shape of the earth (sorry, flat earthers), and can be up to nearly two feet in diameter.

In Competition

Generally, atlas stones are performed in a series. This means multiple stones are loaded onto a platform or over a bar. Oftentimes, the stones are arranged in ascending weight, while the height of the platform or bar descends.

It is becoming increasingly common to see a single weight lifted over a bar (that remains at the same height) for maximum reps in a specific amount of time. For example, you lift a 300-pound stone over a 48-inch bar for a maximum number of reps in 60 seconds. There is also the event of lifting a stone to your shoulder for reps, along with lifting a maximum-weight stone to your shoulder or lifting a maximum-weight stone to a given height.

Technique

Although many people would expect stone lifting to be the epitome of brute power output, good technique is essential when lifting stones.

A personal example by co-author Josh Bryant illustrates the value of good stone-lifting technique. When he began strongman training, he was unable to lift a 220-pound stone. The next week, he trained with professional strongman Odd Haugen, who would go on to become his training partner for two years. With Odd's guidance, Josh lifted a 385-pound stone with ease onto Odd's platform. Stones have a distinct feel and groove, so this is an event that a strong, athletic powerlifter probably won't dominate from day one.

This story is also a testament to Odd's superb coaching.

Now, to refine your stone-lifting techniques, start by rotating the stone to a position where it is motionless. You want the stone to be a particular distance from the platform. Specifically, you want to be close enough to lift the stone onto the platform without having to walk forward, but far enough away so you don't hit the platform when picking up the stone.

In regard to stance, you want to stand with your feet as close as possible while standing over the center of the stone. Spread your hands wide and depress your shoulders (think lats in back pocket). Remember to brace your trunk and your entire upper body. Hinge your body down to the stone, dropping your hands under the center of the stone (as far underneath as you can get them). Wedge your hands hard under the stone. Now, using your forearms, squeeze the stones as hard as you can (as if you are trying to break through the stone with your forearms). While your hips remain at approximate deadlift height, produce force through the ground and pick up the stone. As the stone lifts off the ground, slightly narrow your stance with a little shuffle to get the stone to your lap.

Pull the stone onto your lap. Remember, it needs to be tight to your body, the closer the better!

The stone will be pinned against you in that chest to sternum area. Ideally, you can place your arms from here over the top of the stone. But the next best position is to wrap your arms around the stone (this develops substantial wrestling/grappling isometric clinch/constriction strength). From the lapped position, drive your hips forward while simultaneously pulling the stone back into you. The final movement is to drive up into a full triple extension and load the stone on the platform.

Training Recommendations

- For technical improvement—four to eight sets, one to five reps, using light weights of 50 to 70 percent of a maximal load, full recovery between sets.
- For maximal strength—two to five sets for one to five reps, full recovery between sets, use 85 to 100 percent of maximal load.
- For hypertrophy—do two to four sets with 65 to 85 percent of maximal loads, for 30 to 60 seconds straight (resting two to three minutes between sets). Focus on executing maximal reps with great technique.
- For overload—pick up a load greater than 100 percent and attempt to set in the lap position.
- In a traditional bodybuilding/powerbuilding split, stone lifting would be performed on a legs or back day.

Beneficial Accessory Movements

The following is a list of beneficial atlas stone accessory movements: deadlifts, deficit deadlifts, stiff-leg deadlifts, stiff-leg deficit deadlifts, front squats, paused front squats, GHR, 45-degree deadlift hyper, Zercher squats, yates rows, Pendlay rows, one-arm dumbbell rows, T-bar prison rows, ab wheel, standing weighted crunches, weighted triple extension movements, dumbbell pause floor fly, kettlebell swings, cable fly, pec deck, and bear hug sandbag carries.

The Atlas Stones in a Program

Day 1	Weight	Rest Interval	Reps	Sets
Log push press rack (cluster set, do one set, rest 15 sec, repeat for 5 minutes)	15 rep max	15 sec	3	??
Hindu push-ups (cluster set, do one set, rest 15 sec, repeat for 5 minutes)	BW	15 sec	5	??
Pull-ups (cluster set, do one set, rest 15 sec, repeat for 5 minutes)	BW	15 sec	1	??
Dumbbell floor pause triceps extension (cluster set, do one set, rest 15 sec, repeat for 5 minutes)	15 rep max	15 sec	5	??
Day 2	**Weight**	**Rest Interval**	**Reps**	**Sets**
Hatfield overload squats	Max weight		5	1
Farmer's walk (cluster set, do one set, rest 15 sec, repeat for 5 minutes)	60%	15 sec	30 feet	??
Backward sled drag, 50 feet (cluster set, do one set, rest 15 sec, repeat for 5 minutes)	70%	15 sec	20 feet	??
One-leg curl	Heavy as possible	90 sec	4	3
Weighted plank, 20 sec	BW + 45	As needed	1	2
Day 3	**Weight**	**Rest Interval**	**Reps**	**Sets**
Face pulls (cluster set, do one set, rest 15 sec, repeat for 5 minutes)	15 rep max	15 sec	12	??
Dips (cluster set, do one set, rest 15 sec, repeat for 5 minutes)	15 rep max	15 sec	4	??
IYT raise	Heavy as possible	45 sec	15	3
Cobra lat pulldowns	Heavy as possible	90 sec	10	3

Day 4	Weight	Rest Interval	Reps	Sets
Deadlift	75%	30 sec	1	10
Stones, 56 inches	80%, 90%, 100%	150 sec	3	3
Hammer curls (cluster set, do one set, rest 15 sec, repeat for 5 minutes)	15 rep max	15 sec	5	??

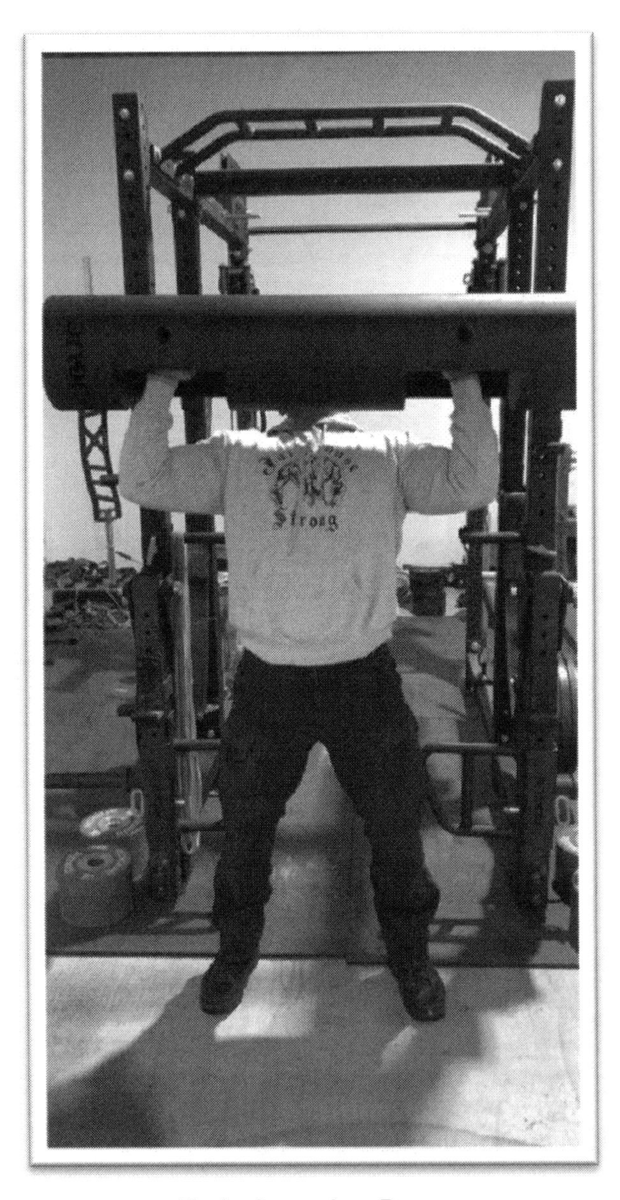

Taylor Lopes Log Press

Log Clean and Press

The log press is the ultimate test of full-body power and upper-body strength!

Logs in competition can range from 8 to 13 inches in diameter and, generally, vary by sex and weight class. Inside of the log are two parallel handles. So, once the log is cleaned, it will be pressed overhead with a neutral grip.

In Competition

Log press can be part of a medley with multiple other events (often pressing ones) for a one-repetition maximum or maximum reps at a preordained weight. Depending on the specifics of the particular event, the most weight lifted, the most reps completed, or the fastest time wins the most points in the log clean and press.

Technique

The first thing you want to do is prevent a possible injury. So, if there are no plates on the log, place the ends on tires so you don't smash your toes.

Now, tilt the log slightly away from you. You want the handles facing forward because this helps with rotation and elbow position when executing the clean portion of the lift.

In regard to stance, place your feet hip – to shoulder-width apart. Hinge down to the log. From here, place your hands on the handles, and you are set in position to deadlift the log. Lift the log to your hip crease and drop down into the lap position, keeping the log in tight to your body.

Now, in one sequential burst, explode upward, driving your elbows under and around while the log remains tight to your body. Extend your hips (some even think about throwing the head back) and clean the log to the rack position. It's now time to press the log! Your lats should be flared and your elbows up. Squeeze your glutes and brace your trunk. The log should be sitting right under your chin. In an instant, dip down with your hips and knees while keeping your elbows up into approximately a quarter squat position. Drive up out of this position, push pressing the log, and driving your head through to lockout.

Training Recommendations

- For technical improvement—four to eight sets, one to five reps, using light weights of 50 to 70 percent of a maximal load, full recovery between sets.
- For maximal strength—two to five sets for one to five reps, full recovery between sets, use 85 to 100 percent of maximal load.
- For hypertrophy—do two to four sets with 65 to 85 percent of maximal loads, for 30 to 60 seconds straight (resting two to three minutes between sets). Focus on executing maximal reps with great technique.
- For overload—do a reverse band technique in the power rack (removing the clean portion).
- In a traditional bodybuilding/powerbuilding split, the log clean and press would be performed on a pressing, shoulder, or upper-body day.

Beneficial Accessory Movements

The following is a list of beneficial log clean and press movements: overhead press, overhead press against bands, reverse band overhead press, dips, close-grip bench press, incline press, Z press, overhead dicks press, JM press, safety bar JM press, front squat static holds, swiss bar curls, any triceps isolation movement, hammer curls, log cleans, log press, and partial rack lockouts.

The Log Clean and Press in a Program

Day 1

Exercise	Sets	Reps/Distance	Rest Interval	Weight/Intensity
Speed Log Clean and Press	10	3	60 sec	50%
Neutral-Grip Pull-Ups	3	8	60 sec	Maximum
Seal Rows	3	12	60 sec	Maximum
Overhead Dicks Press	4	8	60 sec	Maximum
Hammer Curls	3	15	45 sec	Maximum

Day 2

Exercise	Sets	Reps/Distance	Rest Interval	Weight/Intensity
Front Squats	3	3	As needed	3-rep max
Farmer's Walk	4	40 feet	As needed	Maximum
GHR	4	4	60 sec	Maximum
Backward Sled Drag	6	50 feet	60 sec	Maximum
Front Squat Static Holds	2	15 sec	60 sec	Maximum

Day 3

Exercise	Sets	Reps/Distance	Rest Interval	Weight/Intensity
Axle Overhead Press	3	1	As needed	Find new max
Lat Pulldowns	3	12	60 sec	Maximum
Close-Grip Floor Press	3	3	180 sec	Maximum
Incline Rolling Dumbbell Triceps Extension	3	15	45 sec	Maximum
Viking Press	1	Maximum	N/A	50%

Day 4

Exercise	Sets	Reps/Distance	Rest Interval	Weight/Intensity
Speed Zercher Squats	12	2	45 sec	50%
Atlas Stones	4	4	90 sec	60%
Keg Throws	12	1	25 sec	
Leg Press	15	2	45 sec	Maximum
Leg Curls	15	3	15 sec	15-rep max

The movements described above are the four base events. Here are the Cliffs Notes versions of some other fairly common events.

- ***Tire flips:*** If you want to develop explosive strength, this is the rich man's power clean! Do 6 to 15 singles with 30-second breaks between sets. Use a light to moderate weight so you can focus on generating explosive power. For strength, do sets of one to five reps with heavy weight. Take a full recovery between sets, and do two to four sets. For muscle hypertrophy, do three to five sets of four to eight repetitions with moderately heavy weight, and rest 90 to 180 seconds between sets. These should be performed as part of your squat or deadlift workout or on a separate events day. Tire flips build explosive power, work capacity, and bear wrasslin' strength. In Josh's entire strength career, he has had one acute injury, a torn biceps, and this happened flipping a 1,400-pound tire. Always make sure you have a seasoned strongman teach you how to do any event. KEEP YOUR ARMS STRAIGHT while flipping a tire; biceps tears are the injury most commonly associated with tire flips. Realize that these have a high reward, but are also high risk.

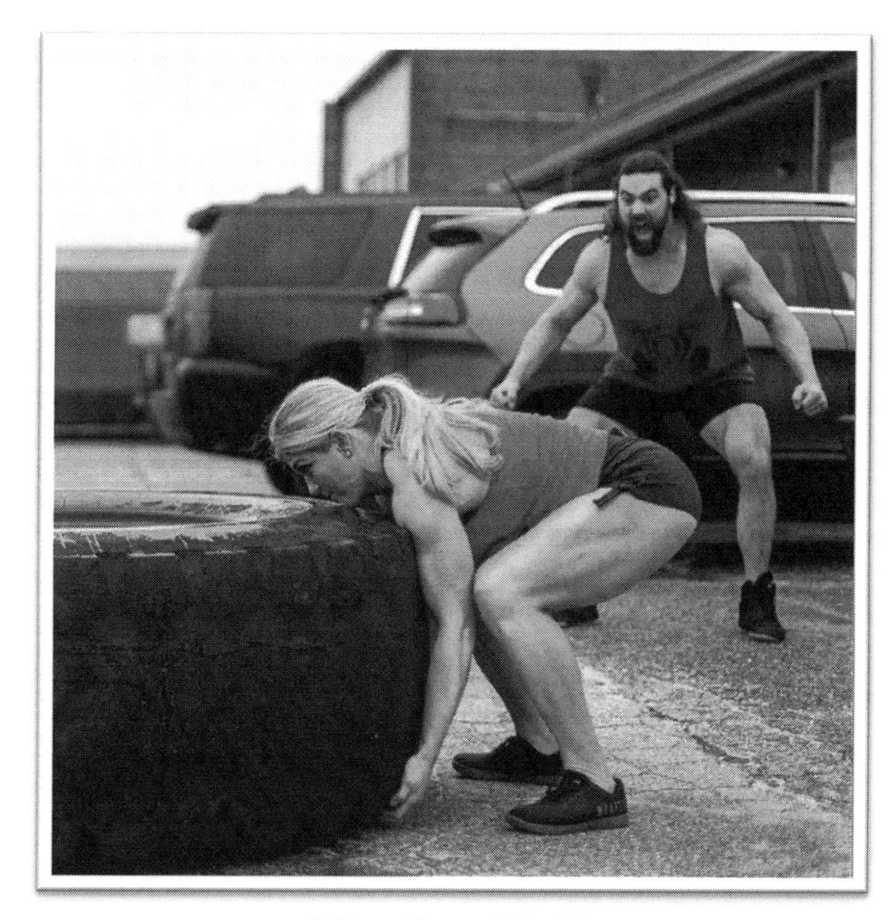

Brittany Diamond Tire Flip

- ***Viking press:*** Viking presses are a great way to build explosive power and pack slabs of beef on your upper body. For explosive power, do one to three reps for 5 to 12 sets with 50 percent of your one-rep maximum. Rest 45 seconds between sets. For strength, use fewer than five repetitions with greater than 85 percent of your one-rep maximum, taking a full recovery between sets. For hypertrophy, do 6 to 15 reps for two to five sets, taking breaks of 90 to 180 seconds between sets. This is best done on a shoulders day or a pressing day. It can also be done on a separate events day.

- ***Crucifix hold:*** Do two or three sets for 60 to 90 seconds. Start with light dumbbells or kettlebells (5 to 15 pounds) in each hand. This is a great exercise for building strength, endurance, shoulder size, and metaphorical testicles. Crucifix holds should be performed on your shoulders day or pressing day. They can also be done on a separate events day.

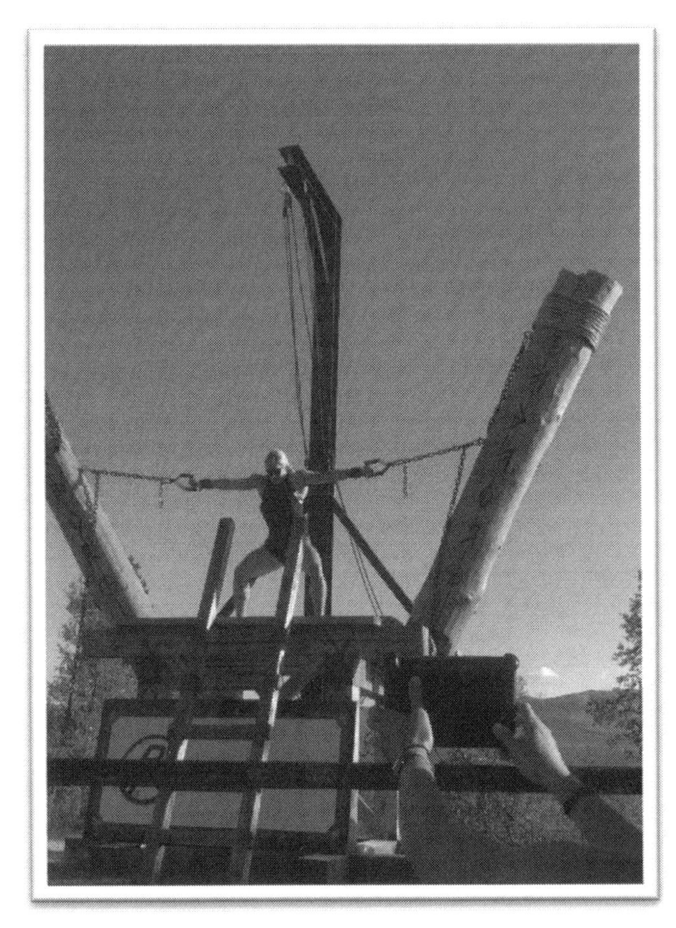

Brittany Diamond Hercules Hold

- ***Truck pulls:*** This event will add herculean size and strength to your back and biceps while working your entire body! Instead of focusing on distance, pull for 30 to 45 seconds with maximum effort, and then take a full recovery. Repeat two or three times. These should be performed on your deadlift day or on a separate events day. Generally, in strongman contests, the duration of a truck pull is 30 to 60 seconds. Staying inside of that time frame will help you mimic a contest, and this is also a good duration if you desire a "Chippendales' ready physique."
- ***Keg rolls:*** These are an excellent exercise for building explosive power! If this is your goal, do one to five reps for three to six sets with a moderately light weight and focus on the speed of the movement. Rest 45 to 60 seconds between sets. For strength, follow the same sets and reps but use a heavier keg. For hypertrophy, do 6 to 15 reps for three or four sets and rest 90 to 180 seconds. This should be performed as part of your squat or deadlift workout or on a separate events day. Remember, kegs are not difficult to get. Most beer joints or liquor stores will give you a free keg.

- ***Sled drags:*** This is one of the greatest movements for muscle hypertrophy of the quads. "Mirror monkeys" should be on these like white on rice! Drag a sled backward for 50 to 100 feet for multiple sets with a maximum weight. Your quads will experience an anerobic burn contrasted to a night in purgatory with leg extension drop sets. To work the hamstrings and glutes, pull the sled forward, with the apparatus dragging behind you. Rest one to two minutes between sets and do 4 to 10 sets. Do this on your squat day or on a separate events day. This can also be a very effective active recovery method. The day after you squat or do events that tax your lower body, do multiple trips with 10 to 25 percent of a max sled weight for 50 to 100 yards. This will serve as an efficient active recovery and help build your work capacity. The sled is also an effective method for strengthening the thighs and posterior chain without the spinal loading of a squat or deadlift. This can allow you to give your back a break while giving your legs a blast. The Finns claim that their deadlift prowess is in large part because of dragging trees backward like a sled as part of their work.

Final Thoughts

If you want functional strength with direct transference to a plethora of real-world scenarios, start training strongman events.

Look, when you apply strength in real-world situations, it's not an evenly balanced barbell sitting in front of you. The situations could be as varied as helping your new Tinder fling move a couch up a flight of stairs or your boss at the fusion restaurant where you work initiating a dollar sake night and now you have to drag inebriated bodies out the door. Whatever the situation, strongman training in all its unorthodox glory will build the kind of muscle you need to complete the task before you.

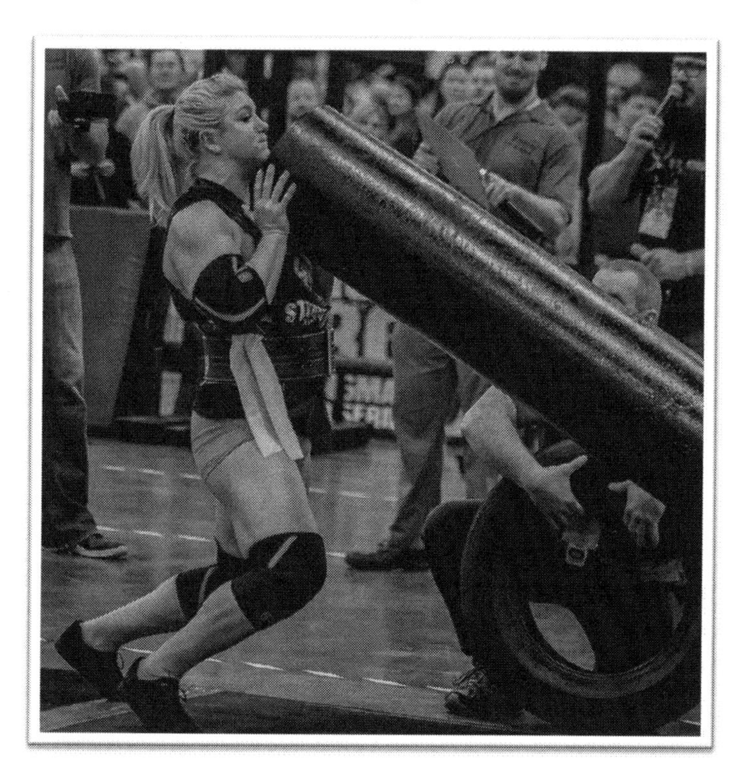

Brittany Diamond Ready for Anything

Strongman is training for real life. You now have the information to make strongman events benefit you.

THE COMMERCIAL GYM AND STRONGMAN TRAINING

Over time, a pattern became established. We went to the gym, trained hard, and after our sessions, we'd go check out what Thic Vic was doing over on his personalized outdoor training deck. While this outside area was part of the commercial gym, a portion of the space was really customized to his specifications.

Once he finished his workout, Vic would take our questions and pass on his insights on a wide range of topics from functional conditioning to situational awareness. He also gave us some advice on dating.

For instance, he would tell us that a "slow dime was better than a fast nickel." This meant that when it came to relationships, you needed to understand that a quality partner was someone in whom you needed to invest time and energy. If you wanted to settle for someone of lesser value, then you needn't worry about making a more significant investment.

It became pretty clear that Thic Vic and his training methods were distinct from the rest of the gym.

So, one day, we asked him, "Thic Vic, why are you training at a commercial gym?"

He gave a deep guttural roar of a chuckle.

"You mean, if I'm not on the 'good girl/bad girl' machine, what am I doing here?" He gestured toward the hip adductor machine, which at that moment was being used by Candi from the local adult cabaret.

"Yeah, I guess that's what we're wondering."

"Look guys, I'm blue collar through and through. But I got my dreams of one day owning some property, with a full-sized garage. Now, when that day comes," he pointed aggressively with his index finger as if to indicate that indeterminate moment in the future, "I will fill my garage rim to rim with all the best strongman training tools.

"In the meantime," his voiced dropped a little as if he resigned himself to the reality of his current situation, "I'm in a small apartment. I don't have close to enough room for everything I need.

"But I got some contract gigs I'm lining up over in the Middle East. Once they come through, I'll have enough dough to set myself up with my own premier garage facility." Vic said this with such excitement and pride.

"Is there another gym around here that could offer you a better environment for strongman training?"

"No, not really. Look, guys, there aren't a lot of people who are training like this." This was the 1990s, well before sleds, battle ropes, and other forms of unorthodox strength training were common features at most gyms.

"So I make the most of where I am and what I have."

Thic Vic embodied the *Jailhouse Strong* philosophy.

How to Train for Strongman at a Commercial Gym

As we've discussed, the functional, demanding movements of strongman benefit far more than the competitive strongman. But what happens when you find yourself in a situation where you don't have access to a quality strongman training facility?

You could find yourself in this situation for any number of reasons. Maybe you don't have the desire, time, or financial resources to buy a bunch of strongman equipment or even the means to drive to the nearest strongman training center. Nonetheless, you can still reap the benefits of strongman training while training at a commercial gym!

Will it be the exact same as training with strongman implements? Will you get every single benefit to the tee? No, but it won't be like kissing your cousin either. So you won't walk away from the experience feeling unfulfilled, slightly morally corrupt, and more than a little uncomfortable.

Basically, at a commercial gym you can get about 80 percent of the strongman training benefits without any of the hassles of driving to a different gym or purchasing strongman equipment.

However, if you plan on competing, we recommend you train on actual strongman implements which best mimic the ones used in competition.

All right, let's take a detailed look at some substitutions you can use at a commercial gym, in the place of strongman equipment.

Overhead Deadlift Hold(s)

Strongman Equivalent: Any grip-related event

Execution: This is a movement we also prescribe to powerlifters to increase deadlift grip strength. Simply, deadlift a bar with a pronated grip (do not use a hook grip), then hold this position for 15 to 30 seconds. Do this for two or three sets at the end of a workout because it destroys your grip and does not leave much for anything else.

Bonus Tip: The more advanced lifter who wants an extreme challenge can do this with two bars simultaneously. This is done by standing with loaded Olympic bars on a rack on both your left and right sides. Set the bars just past arm's length when fully standing up. Be ready for the bars to roll and move around. You will have to keep your grip as you stabilize weight. This will develop your grip and prepare you for grip-focused events. Two or three sets of 15 to 30 seconds are more than enough.

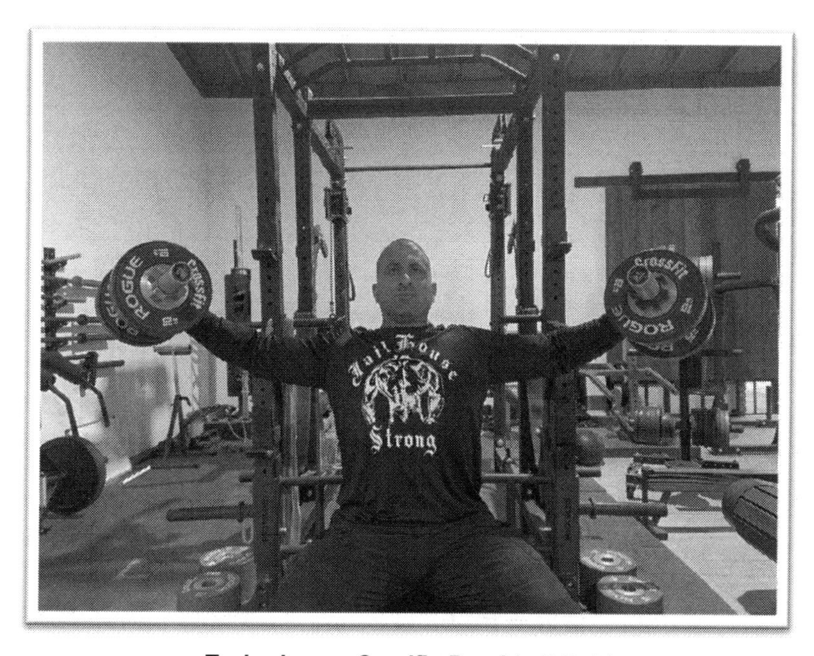

Taylor Lopes Crucifix Dumbbell Hold

Crucifix Dumbbell Hold

Strongman Equivalent: Crucifix Hold

Execution: Set your feet in a shoulder-width stance while maintaining a slight bend in your knees. From here, with your arms fully extended, lift the dumbbells up from your sides and stop when they are parallel to the floor. Hold this position for 30 to 60 seconds for two or three sets. Alternate between a palms-up and palms-down position. Remember, isometric contractions like this are vastly underutilized, so don't be shocked if you start adding extra muscle.

Bonus Tip: If you don't have dumbbells, kettlebells will work great!

Trap Bar Deadlift Farmer's Walk

Strongman Equivalent: Farmer's Walk

Execution: Deadlift the trap bar to lockout. From here, slowly start to walk forward. As you feel comfortable and in control of the weight, you can gradually ***accelerate*** to a brisk pace of walking. Make sure your stepping pattern is even; in training, proper technical execution is much more important than speed. Do three or four sets of 50 to 100 feet. If you run out of room, do not turn with the implement in your hand. Set the weight on the ground; turn around, reset, and repeat. If hypertrophy is the main objective, use straps on this lift. Do not let grip strength limit you.

Bonus Tip: If you do not have a trap bar, heavy dumbbells or even two loaded barbells can be used. Both of these variations are much more difficult than using farmer's walk implements, so weights will need to be reduced.

Zercher Squats

Strongman Equivalent: Conan's Wheel and Zercher Carry Events

Execution: In a squat rack, take a stance where your feet are wider than shoulder width. A fat bar works best, if you have access (a regular barbell is fine, too). Pick the barbell up with the weight in the crook of your arms. From here, execute a squat movement to a depth of parallel or slightly below. Brace hard to hold the position and prevent rounding. Keep the bar in an isometric hold for 15 to 30 seconds. Do two or three sets of three to five reps.

Bonus Tip: Instead of squatting the barbell (while holding in the Zercher position), walk in place with it for 15 to 30 seconds, for two or three sets. This even more closely mimics the demands of a Zercher carry or Conan's Wheel.

One-Arm Cable Rope Row

Strongman Equivalent: Truck Pull (hand over hand)

Execution: With a rope attachment at chest level, you will be standing facing a cable stack. Stand with good posture and with your feet slightly wider than shoulder-width apart. With your arm fully extended, grab the rope with one hand. Place your other hand at waist level. From here, powerfully and quickly pull the rope toward your midsection while slightly rotating your body. Remember to get your hips into the movement. Pause briefly at the completed position, then return to the start position. Repeat this for 10 to 15 reps before alternating sides. Do two or three sets on each side.

Bonus Tip: You can also perform this movement on a seated row for the exact same set and rep prescription.

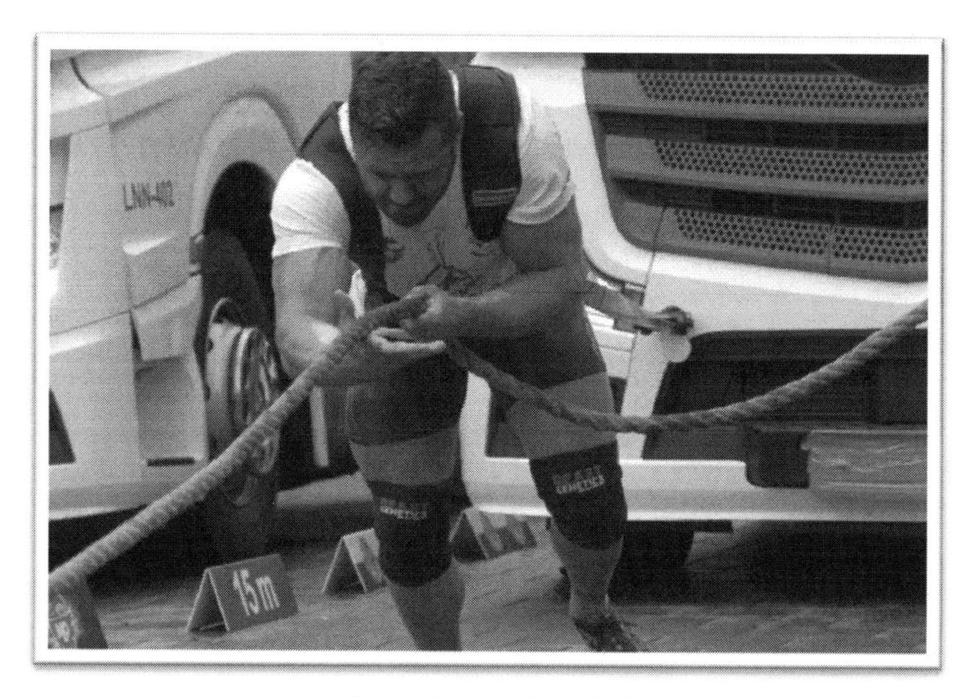

Tyson Morrissy Truck Pull

Plate Loads

Strongman Equivalent: Atlas Stones

Execution: Preferably, get a loading pin. If you don't have access to one, you can unscrew the pin sleeve of a cheap barbell (commercial gyms always have these). From here, load plates on the sleeve/pin. When available, bumper plates are best. Make sure that the plates are standing up, so the pin/sleeve will be on its side. From here, approach the apparatus and line up your big toe with the center position of the plate. Now, with an approximate shoulder-width stance, spread your fingers apart as wide as you can so you have more surface area to grab the plates; from here, put yourself down into a position where your shoulders are over the plates. Then squeeze the plates and pull them up in a straight line to triple extension. This can be done in one motion, or by lapping the plates in a squatted position before extending up. Do this for two or three sets of three to five reps.

Bonus Tip: When you have no loading pin, you can do the plate stack row. You place a stack of 45-pound plates on top of a 10-pound plate, so you can get your fingers underneath. Straddle the stack so your feet are right outside the plates and your toes are in line with the plate holes. From here, with slightly bent knees, grab the plate stack with your fingers underneath, palms against the side, and forearms squeezing the stack. Now row the plates to your chest. Do this for two or three sets of six to eight reps.

Backward Sled Drags

Strongman Equivalent: Any Backward Sled Drag

Execution: Now that many commercial gyms have sleds, we had to include this movement. "Backward" simply means that you are facing the sled and pulling it backward. Lean backward with your arms straight and pull away from the sled with maximum intensity; if this looks like a relaxing back pedal, add more weight. Never let the sled stop. Use your bodyweight to lean away from the sled throughout the entire movement; never row the weight. Pull it with your body. Keep in mind that your arms are the weak link, not your legs. Think of your arms as "hooks" that do not move. Take fast, short, choppy steps, unlike traditional sprints. Long strides will slow you down. Since you should be going heavy, force exertion is critical; you will apply more force with small steps. Do four to six sets of 50 to 150 feet.

Bonus Tip: The sled is a very versatile piece of equipment. You can use it as resistance to sprint forward or attach a rope to it and do arm over arm pulls. The possibilities are endless.

Squat Rack Viking Press

Strongman Equivalent: Viking Press

Execution: Place two barbells across a power rack, with the barbells resting on the safety bar. The safety bars on the side in which you will be pressing, however, should be four to six inches lower than the stationary end. On the stationary end of the barbell, place two 10-pound plates both pushing against the safety bar (one plate outside the safety bar, the safety bar in the middle, and one plate inside the safety bar); this will prevent the apparatus from sliding as you press. From the pressing side of the apparatus (outside of the power rack), execute 8 to 12 reps for two or three sets.

Bonus Tip: Cheap, effective Viking Press attachments can be purchased online.

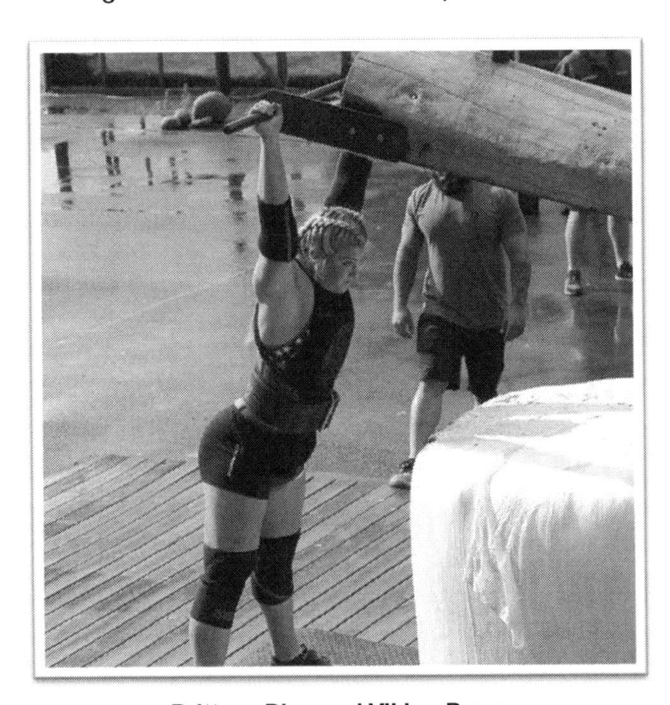

Brittany Diamond Viking Press

Trap Bar Jumps

Execution: Start in the same way as a trap deadlift. But instead of locking out at the top, explosively jump as high as you can. Make sure to keep your arms straight and avoid pulling up with your hands. Focus on jumping as high as possible. To avoid injury, it's crucial to pay attention to your landing. Land softly; absorb the force from the jump and the added weight by landing on the balls of your feet. Remember to push your hips back, keep your back flat, and prevent your knees from collapsing together. Reset between each rep, and do one to three reps for three to five sets.

Bonus Tip: Studies show these are superior to Olympic lifts for power production for regular athletes. Power production peaks between 20 and 30 percent of a one-rep max. So there is no reason to ever go heavy on these!

Bonus Section

Tires/Kegs

Strongman contests often include tire flipping. These tires weigh anywhere from a few hundred pounds to well over a thousand, depending on the level.

While some regular gyms now have tires, a vast majority do not. Nonetheless, you can easily access tires with just a little ingenuity.

Did you know that it costs dumps and tractor supply companies a lot of money to dispose of their large tires? This means that they are extremely easy to find and they are free! A quick Google search will offer plenty of locations where tractor tires are sold. With that information, you will be good to go! As long as you have somewhere to store your tire, like a garage, backyard, or even a front yard (so long as no HOA is involved), you can have a tire or tires at no cost to you.

What about kegs? Most bars will give you an empty keg for free. In some cases, they may charge a very nominal fee (a price less than the day pass of the local commercial gym purgatory).

If you want to leave this keg empty, it will weigh approximately 30 pounds, and you can throw it for height and/or distance. For clean and jerks, you can fill it with water. This will get the weight in the neighborhood of 160 pounds. Filling it with cement can increase the weight to 300-plus pounds. At that point, you could use the keg for loads and rolls. If you use lead shot, the keg will get even heavier.

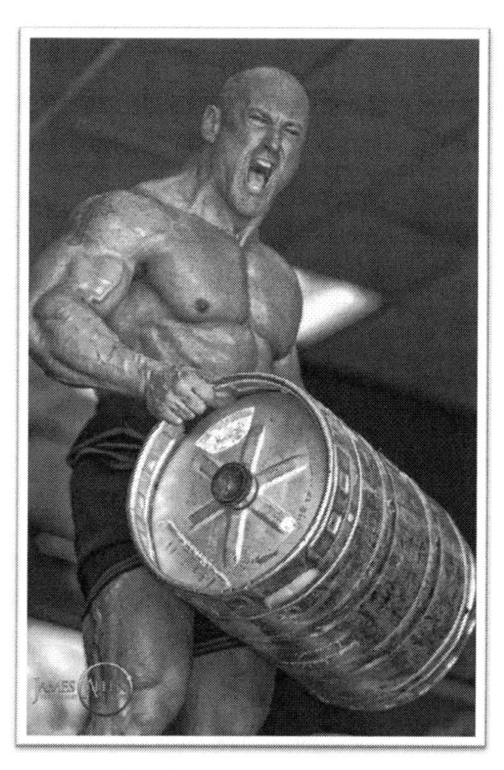

Ed Brown Lifting Kegs

Kegs are great for throws, carries, loads, and rolls; in reality, they're the rainbow coalition of strength training.

No way to get strongman equipment in your tiny apartment garage on Manhattan's Upper East Side? In the words of Pancho Villa, "Don't let it end like this. Tell them I said something."

Don't go quiet into that good night. Find a way to rage, to train, to get strong.

Other Substitutions

While we have provided a detailed breakdown of gym substitutions for strongman events, here is a more extensive, but not exhaustive, list. Remember, necessity is the mother of all invention.

With ingenuity, a lot can get done.

Squatting Events

- Squats
- Front Squats
- Pause Squats
- 1 and ¼ Squats
- Box Squats
- Hack Squats
- Smith Machine Squats
- Dead Squats
- Goblet Squats
- Bodyweight Squats

Deadlift Events

- Deadlift
- Smith Machin Deadlifts
- Trap Bar Deadlifts
- Rack/Block Deadlifts (partial ROM from various heights)
- Deficit Deadlifts
- Trap Bar Deadlifts
- Snatch Grip Deadlifts
- Barbell Hack Squats
- Dumbbell Deadlifts

Clean and Press Events/Press Events

- Clean and Press (barbell & dumbbell)
- Clean and Push Press (barbell & dumbbell)
- Clean and Jerks (barbell & dumbbell)
- Standing One-Arm Dumbbell Press (off arm braced on rack)
- Push Press

- Strict Press
- Z Press
- Machine Overhead Press Variations
- High Pulls
- Power Cleans
- Smith Machine Press
- Dumbbell Press
- Dips
- Close-Grip Bench Press
- Board Press
- Incline Press
- Kettlebell Clean Jerk
- Landmine Press
- OHP/Push Press against Bands
- Partial Lockout OHP
- Barbell Static Holds Overhead at Lockout

Loading/Throwing

- Medicine Ball Throws
- Plate Throws
- High Pulls
- Kettlebell Snatch
- Snatch
- Sandbag Cleans/Loads/Throws
- Swings
- Romanian Deadlifts
- High Pulls (clean or snatch)
- Zercher Squats (regular, paused, or dead)
- Stone Trainer Extensions
- Deadlifts
- Any Triple Extension Movement
- Jumps
- Short Resisted Sprints

Carrying/Dragging

- Unilateral Farmer's Walk (suitcase carry)
- Any Farmer's Walk Variation
- Plate Carries
- Sandbag Carries
- Walking Lunges
- Zercher Carries

- Front Squat Static Hold
- Step-Ups
- Dumbbell Cradle Carries
- Barbell Walks in Place (do in power rack)
- Goblet Carries
- Waiter Walk
- Two-Arm Overhead Carries
- Chain Yoke (Watch our YouTube video on how to make one.)
- Duck Walk (dumbbell, kettlebell, loading pin)
- Stone Trainer Carries

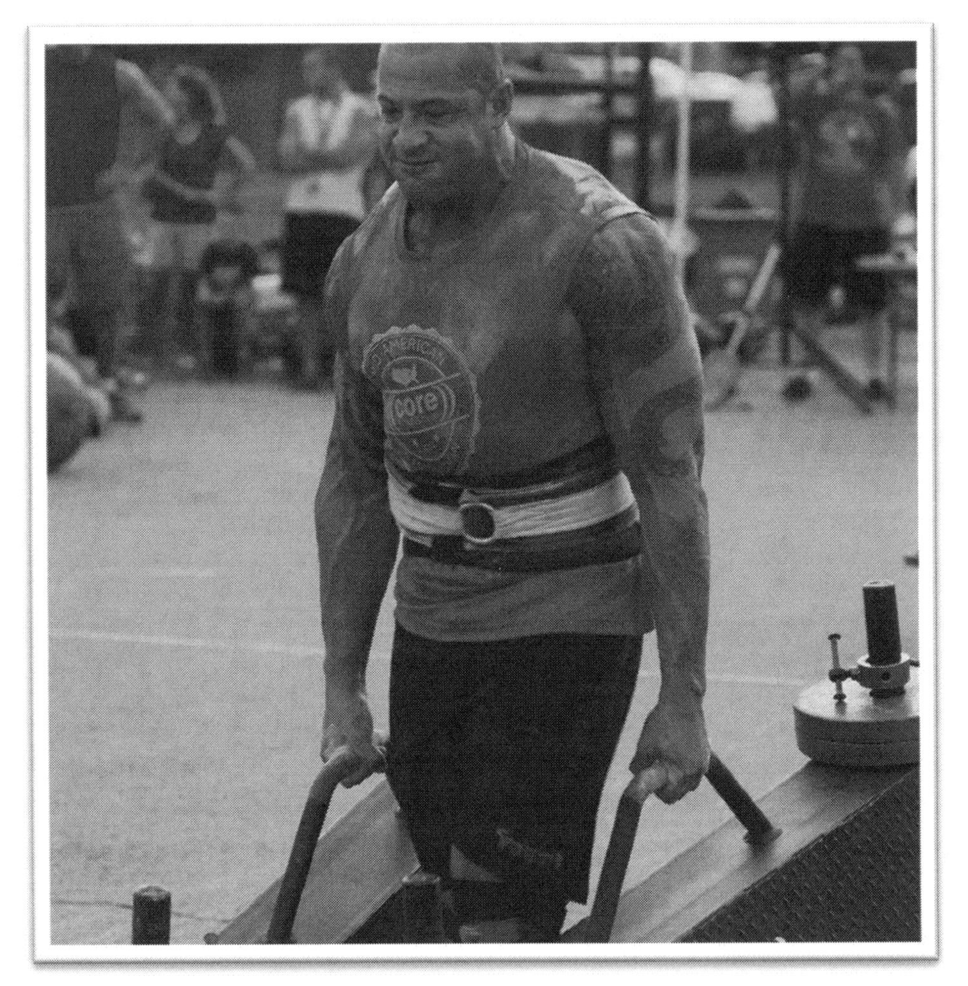

Matt Mills Farmer's Walk

Flipping/Pulling

- Sled Drags
- Dragging any oddly shaped object
- Any Horizontal Pull Exercise
- Any Vertical Pull Exercise

- High Pulls
- Swings
- Throws
- Arm over Arm Pulls (sled/prowler)
- Rope Climbs
- Sled Pulls (attached by weight belt)

Miscellaneous

- Hercules Hold in Cable Crossover
- Crucifix Holds
- Any Deadlift/Farmer Hold
- Hang from a pull-up bar (added weight if applicable)
- Resisted Sprints (sled, hill, sand, etc.)
- Any lift with Fat Gripz added
- Barbell Complexes

Final Thoughts

Admittedly, some of these movements may be an infringement of the commercial gym code of conduct. In regard to this, take the words of G. Gordon Liddy: "Obviously crime pays, or there'd be no crime." Be more concerned about the crime you are committing against yourself by not training strongman events.

Remember the Jailhouse Strong philosophy: Do what you can, with what you have, and where you are!

COMPETING IN STRONGMAN

If you have no interest in ever competing in strongman, feel free to skip over this section.

If you have a slight, passing, general, or intense interest in competing in strongman, read on. In the 1990s and into the 2000s, strongman contests consisted of the promoter's favorite events. This ranged from endurance-happy, CrossFit-like contests, to essentially a powerlifting meet where the log press replaced the bench press, the deadlift had a slightly smaller range of motion, and the squat was lifting as many Hooter's waitresses as possible (they were huddled together on a bizarre apparatus).

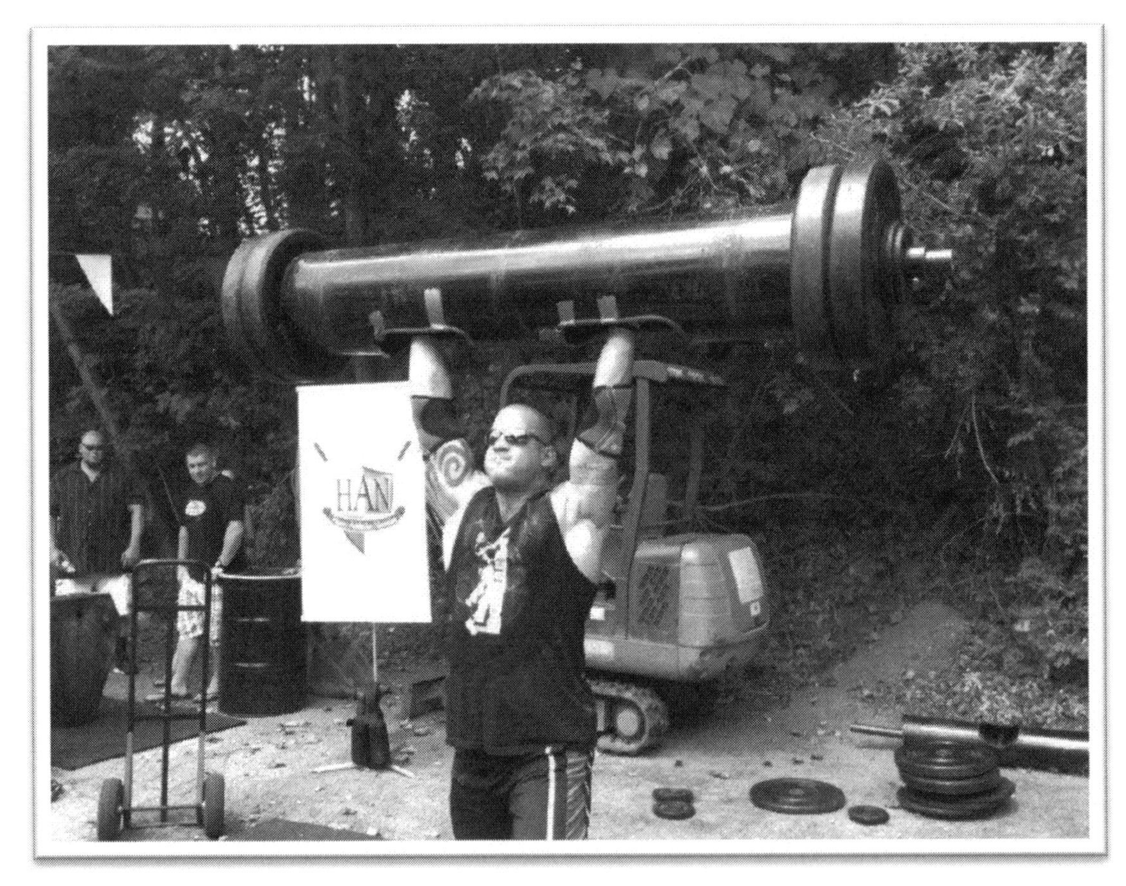

Matt Mills in a Backwoods Strongman Competition

For better or worse, the days of totally randomized events are gone.

While the sport is evolving and becoming more standardized, the strongman competitor still needs to be ready for last-minute changes. Equipment breaks, surfaces become slippery, and implements stored outdoor freeze (we have actually seen this happen). The #GASSTATIONREADY axiom of "stay ready, so you don't have to get ready" is a great mantra for competitive strongman.

Strongman contests can consist of as few as three or four events, but oftentimes five or more, while taking place over one day, two days, or even three days.

The bottom line: Strongman is a sport where the primary objective is to lift unorthodox, heavy objects, and you will often move with these objects. Basically, you lift or lift and move implements of near-maximal weight, and you are scored by the fastest time to completion, the maximum reps completed, or the most weight lifted.

Unlike powerlifting, where all the weight lifted is added together for a total, strongman is scored by points. For example, in a large contest, there may be eight points given per event. Using the log clean and press for an example, the results hypothetically could be as follows:

Pounds Lifted	Placing Points	Awarded
425	1st	8
315	2nd	7
300	3rd	6
295	4th	5
280	5th	4
275	6th	3
270	7th	2
215	8th	1

The way in which the attempts are organized will vary by contest, so it's important for competitors to gather as much information as possible ahead of time and pay attention in the rules briefing. Remember, unlike other competitive strength sports, the events and rules of strongman contests often change on the day of the event.

Additionally, observe the enforcement of the rules with a keen and careful eye. For, example, on a pressing medley event for time, the officials might say, "No dropping implements from overhead." Yet they are letting competitors get away with it. If you don't follow suit, you will lose time and maybe lose the event. When in Rome, do as the Romans do! (For a domestic analogy, remember the Chicago way: You don't bring a knife to a gun fight!)

You also want to be astute in how you go about setting your poundage. In the hypothetical log clean and press for a max (described in the table above), the 425-pound lift clearly dominated the contest. However, no more points were earned than if the same competitor had done 320. Unlike powerlifting where one great lift can "carry" the other mediocre lifts with a large total, the same is not true with strongman; the one-trick pony will never experience success in strongman. After each event is completed, the order of competitors should be rearranged. The rearrangement usually goes as follows: The first-place finisher in the current event will go last in the subsequent event, the second-place finisher will go second to last, the third-place finisher will go third to last, and so on. An additional advantage to winning an event is that you can watch and see what you need to do to win in the subsequent event. If it is an event you dominate, you can be strategic and save energy by completing just what is necessary to win. So, be smart and conserve your strength.

The Strongman Corporation has the following divisions and weight classes:

Heavyweight Men Division

- SHW Class – 300.5# (136.6 kilo) and above
- 300# Class – 264.5# up to 300.4# (136.55 kilo)
- 265# Class – 231.5# (105k) up to 264.5# (120.7 kilo)

Middleweight Men Division

- 200.5# Class (91.14 kilo) to 231.4# (105 kilo)
- 175.5# Class (80 kilo) to 200.4# (91.09 kilo)

Lightweight Men Division

- Up to 150# Class (68 kilo)
- 150.5# Class (68.4 kilo) to 175.4# (79.7 kilo)

Heavyweight Women Division

- 200.5# Class (91.14 kilo) and up
- 180.5# Class (82.05 kilo) to 200.4# (91 kilo)

Middleweight Women Division

- 160.5# Class (72.95 kilo) to 180.4# (82 kilo)
- 140.5# Class (63.86 kilo) to 160.4# (72.91 kilo)

Lightweight Women Division

- 120.5# Class (54.7 kilo) to 140.4# (63.8 kilo)
- Up to 120.4# Class (54.73 kilo)

Furthermore, there are divisions by age, experience, and achievement level. Athletes must be at least 12 years old to compete. Weight classes will differ in different divisions that are organized by experience level, age, and gender.

United States Strongman, a rival federation, classifies athletes beyond weight and gender with the following:

Open: Any athlete who wishes to compete.
Novice: Any athlete who has not competed in an open division or has not won a novice division.
Hero's Division: Police, fire, and military.
Teen: Any athlete between the ages of 13 and 19. (Athletes under the age of 18 must have parental or guardian written consent.)
Masters: 40+, 50+, 60+.

United States Strongman keeps records in the following events, for the above divisions on the state and national level (you can see the corresponding rules for the record to count, next to the event):

1. **Max Log Clean & Press:** 12" log circumference for men, 10" log circumference for women. 60-second time limit per attempt. Three attempts with Wessels Rule (i.e., if you miss any of your attempts, even if it is your first or second attempt, you are done at that point and are credited with the amount of weight you did on the previous attempt). No built-up belts. Feet parallel, knees and elbows locked, head through. No tacky grip allowed.
2. **Max Axle Clean & Press:** 60-second time limit per attempt. Three attempts with Wessels Rule. May not rest on belt. May not launch from belt to rack position. Feet parallel, knees and elbows locked, head through. No tacky grip allowed.*
3. **Max Standard Deadlift:** 60-second time limit per attempt. Three attempts. Wessels Rule applies. Straps and suits allowed. No sumo. Hitching allowed. Hips and knees locked. Down command from the judge.*
4. **Max 18-Inch Deadlift**: 60-second time limit per attempt. Three attempts. Wessels Rule applies. Straps and suits allowed. No sumo. Hitching allowed. 18" measured from the center of the bar to the floor. Hips and knees locked. Down command from the judge.*
5. **Farmer Hold for Time**: Max time. Time starts on lockout and ends when either implement hits the floor.

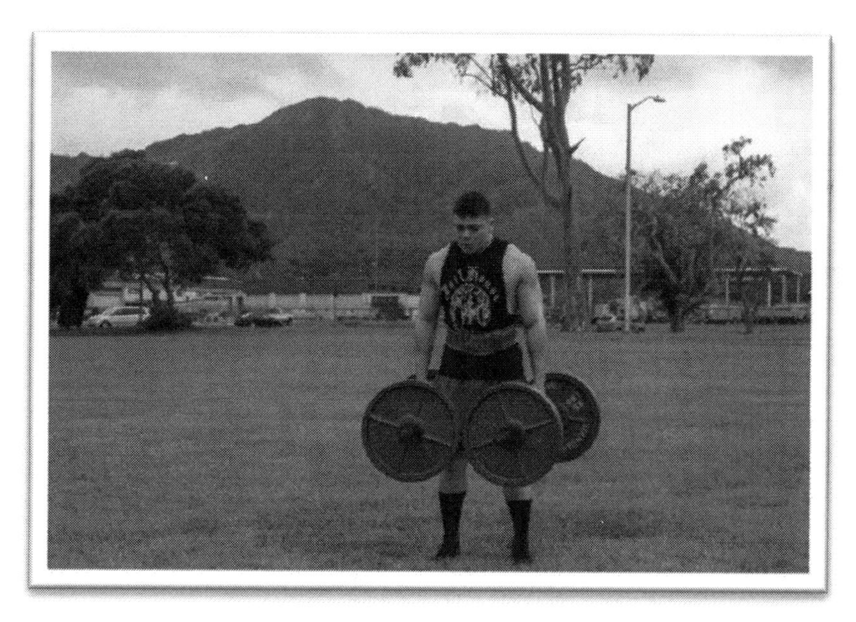

Nick DiLeo Farmer's Walk

Always verify divisions ahead of a contest unless you are fine competing in the open.

Though competitive strongman events are ever changing, there are a number of staples that frequently appear on the international stage, including:

- Atlas Stones
- Axle Press

- Car Flip
- Conan's Wheel
- Deadlift
- Deadlift Hold
- Duck Walk
- Dumbbell Press
- Farmer's Walk
- Fingal's Fingers
- Frame Carry
- Hercules Hold
- Husafell Stone
- Keg Toss
- Loading Race
- Log Clean and Press
- Power Stairs
- Squat
- Tire Flip
- Vehicle Pull
- Viking Press
- Yoke Carry

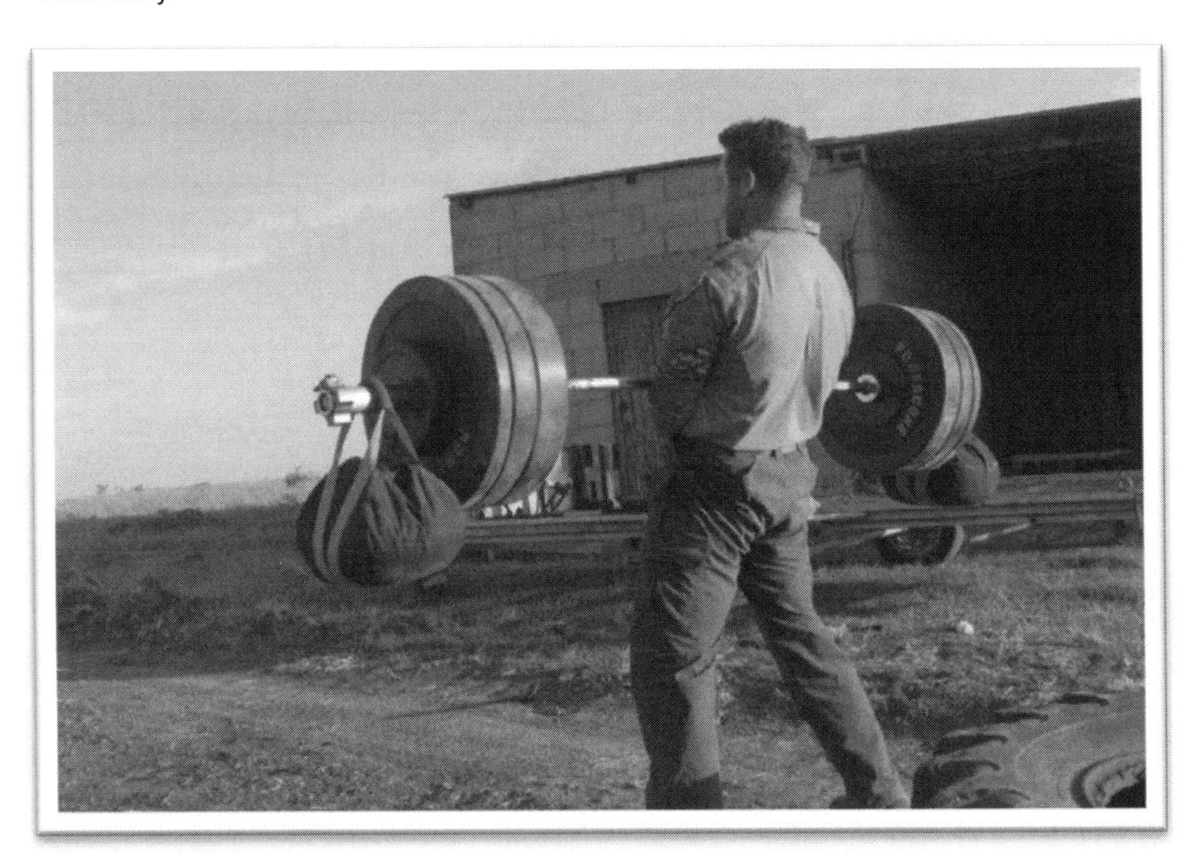

Harry Walker Front Carry in the Middle of a Deserted Tundra

These events are common ones, but many promoters still love to throw events out of left field, so be ready. A medley is simply a combination of two or more events.

Final Thoughts

Strongman is for everyone! If you want to compete, there is a division for you. Don't hesitate to pull the trigger! This is not MMA or backyard boxing; no one will physically harm you during the competition. You only have to overcome your toughest challenge: the reality created in the six inches between your ears. While emancipation from mental limitations is not easy, it is achievable.

For more info on competing in strongman, go to:

United States Strongman: https://www.unitedstatesstrongman.com/

Strongman Corporation: https://www.strongmancorporation.com/

Entering a Strongman Contest

So, it's the middle of the night. You're in the midst of a cross-country road trip to start a new gig on the opposite coast. After driving for 18 hours, you're just trying to find a secluded place to catch some quick shut-eye. You pull up to some little bitty, run-down, deserted Conoco gas station. Sleep comes quickly. But then you wake up with a start. Your car is surrounded by some of the rastiest dudes you've ever seen. Turns out you're in the middle of a Freight Train Riders of America (FTRA) hobo war party camp. These guys want your cash and your ride.

Rest easy. You know that you will confidently handle the situation because of strongman training. Remember, strongman training is real-life training.

The only thing is that all of your strongman training has got you hooked on training endorphins, and now you're looking to take the feeling to the next level with competitive strongman.

Great, we are here to help.

We have compiled 14 tips for a successful first strongman competition. These are not just for competitors. They can also be used by the weekend warrior or anyone who wants to maximize their performance with strongman events.

See a Strongman Contest Up Close and Personal: You can read all the strongman articles you want. You could also fall down a YouTube "rabbit hole," watching strongman contests. But it's not the same as going to one! If you are able to do it, attend a strongman contest before you compete in one. Strongman contests have a distinct feel. Experience that feeling before you compete.

Rest and Supplements: During the week leading up to the contest, make sure you're well rested (skip those sleepless, 90-proof nights). During that week, cut back on the stimulants. Not only will you sleep better, but when you take your favorite pre-workout on the day of the contest, it'll feel like the first time all over. You'll be a raging bull ready to take the platform. Do your best to stick with your normal morning routine. If you normally have a light breakfast, don't slam two All-Star breakfasts at Waffle House. This is especially true the day of the contest. If your diet resembles Morgan Spurlock's "Super-Size Me" experiment, super-size yourself into the contest, don't go all "farm to table" two days out. Experimenting with any unfamiliar foods or supplements risks an adverse reaction!

The Rules of the Game: For a max log lift, you may get three attempts. Or you may get unlimited attempts and are only "out" after two misses. You may be allowed drops on the farmer's walk, or you may not be. Is tacky grip spray allowed on the stones? Can you drop the axle from overhead on the axle press, yoke, or anchor drag medley? Okay, you get the idea.

Know the rules of the contest by paying attention during the rules briefing. Also observe the *enforcement* of rules. For instance, if dropping the axle from overhead is against the rules *but* it's not being enforced, you can be a martyr in Rome or a Roman in Rome.

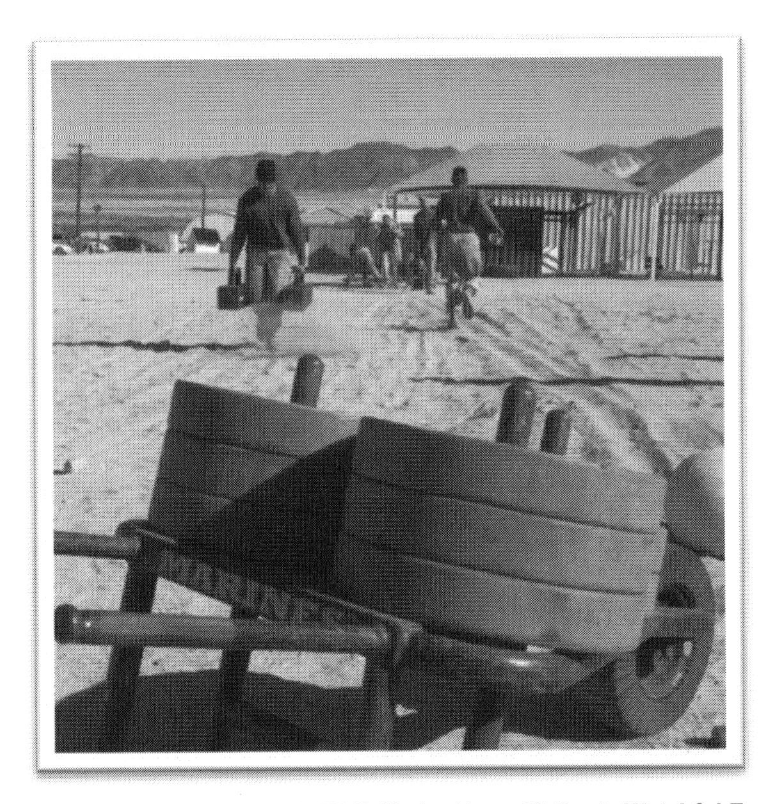

Marines Perform a Farmer's Walk Under Harry Walker's Watchful Eye

Compete at Your Training Weight: In elite-level, professional athletics, weight cuts are the norm. But does it really make sense to cut weight for a contest in the local Hooter's parking lot? Your first strongman contest should be a fun learning experience where your energy is devoted to event proficiency and gaining strength. Strongman competitor Chris Vachio says, "If the number of competitions you have done is less than the amount of weight you need to cut, don't do it." By restricting fluids and calories you are adding another dimension of stress. It is *not a good idea* for your first contest. As you gain experience, we suggest cutting weight only for elite-level competitors for very important contests. Go out and have fun!

Gym Bag Check: There is nothing more stressful than showing up to a contest and forgetting an important piece of gear. The day before you leave for your contest, completely empty your gym bag and repack while doing an inventory check along the way. Make a paper or digital checklist of what you need ahead of time and check items off one by one as you repack your gym bag.

This action will prevent last-minute scrambling and stress.

Be Strong Enough: How strong is strong enough? This depends on the contest. It does not feel good to score a zero on an event or get crumpled by a weight. If your deadlift max is 500 pounds, max yoke for 50 feet is 585 pounds, and max log press is 255 pounds, would it make sense to do a contest with a 650-pound deadlift for reps, an 800-pound yoke, and a 300-pound log for reps? Strong enough is relative. Challenge yourself, but be realistic.

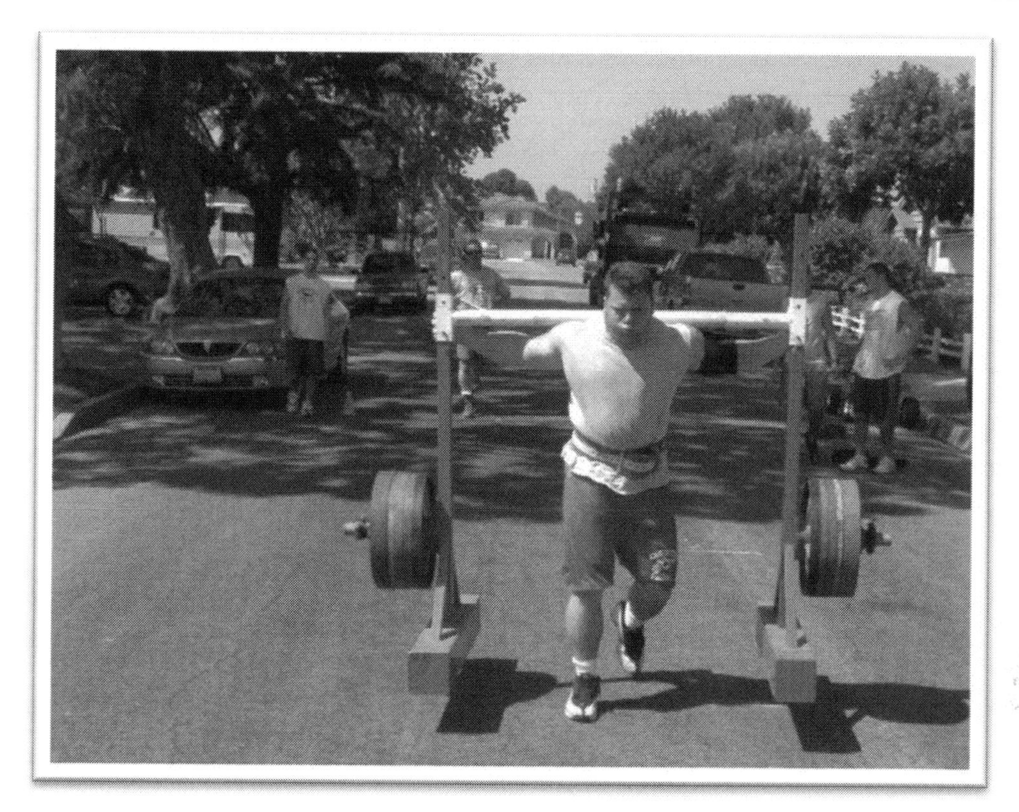

Author Josh Bryant Yoke – 2003

Adequate Conditioning: Some powerlifters achieve great success on the platform but get winded walking up a flight of stairs or in the midst of an "intimate encounter." Limit strength is your base, but you must also have the lung capacity to go all out for 60 seconds. This is accomplished with your specific event training, not endless hours on the treadmill. Strength is the name of the game, but many events will require you to execute grueling max reps or medleys that combine multiple events. Additionally, by being conditioned, not only will you be more gas station ready in a possible self-defense scenario and Chippendales ready for a neighborhood pool party, but you will recover more quickly between training days, training exercises, and events on the day of the contest.

Train Events (Preferably with Competitors): Strength centers that have strongman implements are popping up like pills at a Charlie Sheen party. The website "Starting Strongman" has a gym finder that will help you locate where you can find gyms with strongman equipment.

The strongman community is very welcoming. If you show up with a good attitude to a strongman gym, competitors will often help you with advice and technical cues. Familiarizing yourself with strongman implements will greatly help you on contest day.

Have the Right Shoes: This, in large part, comes down to a personal preference, how serious you are about competing, and your finances. Matt Mills, whom we interviewed for the book and a long-time client of co-author Josh Bryant, had the following recommendations. For pressing, a squat shoe works well because it can help keep you more upright when you dip to use your legs and it offers more stability in the heel. The same rationale applies to power stairs. For heavy carrying events, Matt recommends hiking shoes because of the support and the ability to still move fast. For heavy yokes, do not wear cushy running shoes or you will be extremely unstable when you move. For deadlifting, wearing socks or deadlift slippers keeps you closest to the ground. However, some people prefer wrestling shoes, while others like powerlifting-specific deadlift shoes. For truck pulls or other similar events, rock climbing shoes are hands down the recommended footwear.

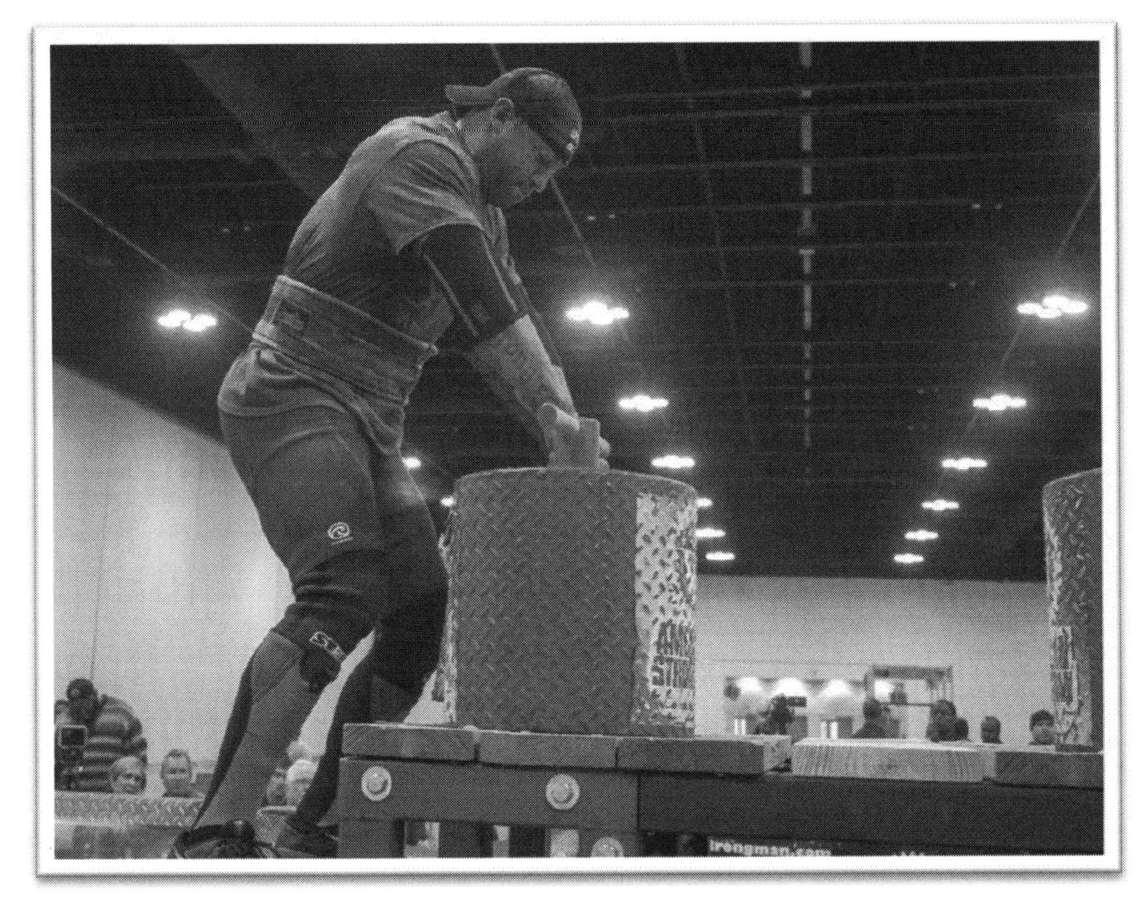

Matt Mills Performs Power Stairs

Other Miscellaneous Gear: We recommend a 13 mm power belt, high-quality wrist wraps, wrist straps, elbow sleeves, knee sleeves, knee wraps, a squat suit, and a deadlift suit. With all of these pieces of equipment purchased from reputable brands, you will have everything you ever need to establish your competitive strongman prowess.

Save Your Best for the Contest: Every event in training, every set and rep you do, is not going to be a PR. Grinding out a yoke PR that takes four minutes and 53 seconds, with 14 drops along the way, five days out from a contest might feel like progress. But this type of overly ambitious training will have serious consequences come meet day. Training is for building strength and event mastery. Strongman contests are for demonstrating it!

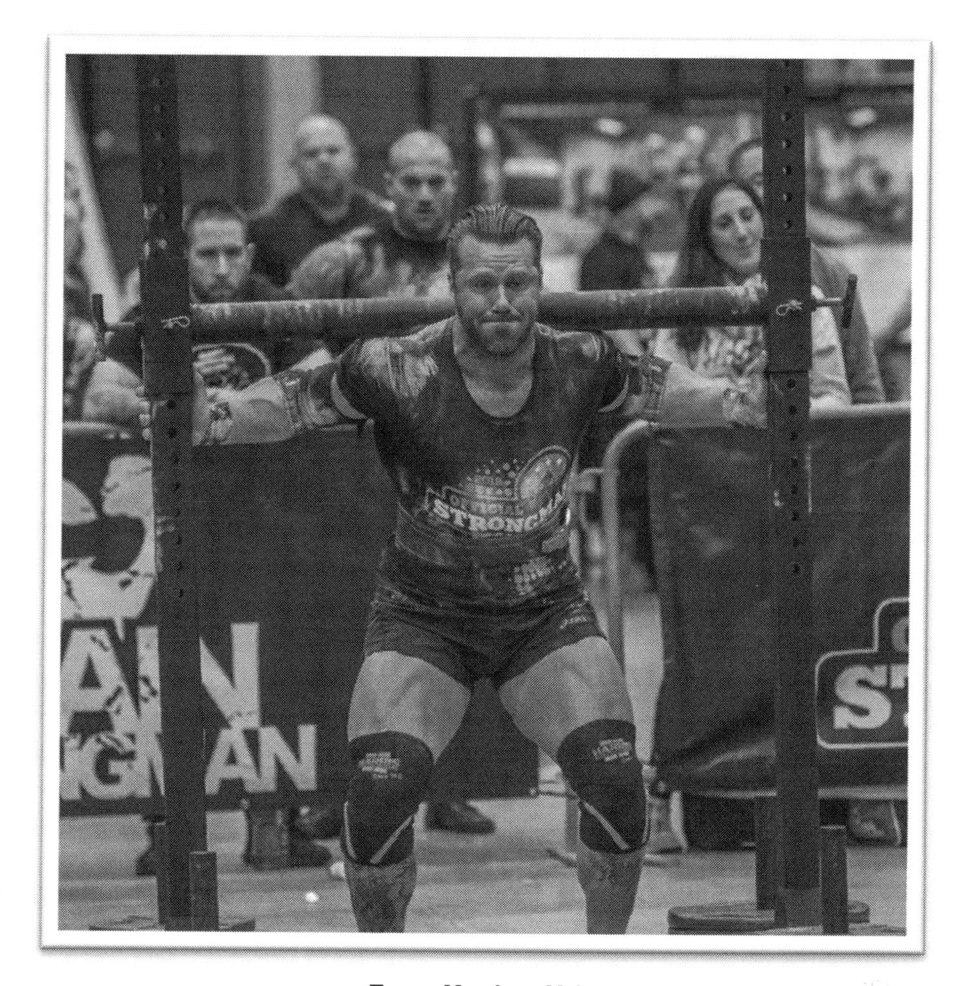

Tyson Morrissy Yoke

Eat and Stay Hydrated: Most strongman competitions have five-plus events, and each event can take up to a couple hours. Frequently, these contests are outdoors during summer months.

Even when you are just standing outside, hydration would be an issue. It is that much more of an issue over the course of a day with multiple maximal-exertion events. We recommend eating light foods like meal replacement bars, fruits, potatoes, and pasta. Keep protein sources lean, and hydrate with Gatorade and water. Do not experiment with foods the day of the event. Opt for the safe bet!

Do Not Ejaculate during Contest Week (Men Only): The old-time prize fighting coaches weren't stiffs. They were spot on! You will be like a rabid dog contest day, if you have the discipline to avoid "getting off" by staying on target with your goals. There is some interesting research on the relationship between ejaculation and serum testosterone level in men. Regardless of test levels, the psychological aggressiveness from the spartan tactic will have you eating lightning and crapping thunder on contest day. This approach can be related to the concept of sexual transformation, or the process of converting sexual energy into some other drive, motivation, or energy of a higher order.

Freddy Fear Your Friend, Nerves: We can tell you from our experiences competing in strongman and other high-level athletic competitions: It's totally normal to feel nervous at a strongman contest. As long as you don't let it overwhelm you, being in this mental state can actually fuel your performance. Stay as relaxed as possible, until it's time to go. Ask your coach or training partner to hang out with you to help you stay calm and reduce your anxiety. Breathing deeply and meditating have both worked to calm our nerves.

Strongman Standards

The requisite level of strength required to enter a strongman contest depends on the contest. They are all different. Michael Gill, world class masters strongman competitor and coach, offered the following tables of lifts to be considered a well-rounded strongman competitor and do well in a national or professional contest in the listed weight categories.

Lifting Standards—Ladies

	140	140 Pro	180
Log Max	130	150	170
Log Reps	120/6	135/6	160/6
Yoke 75 Feet (no drops, under 15 seconds)	400	450	500
Farmer's Walk 75 Feet (no drop sub 20 sec)	165	185	200
Cement Stone	200	250	280
Cement Stone (8 reps in 60 sec)	175	200	220
Deadlift Max	315	350	405

	180 Pro	Open	Open Pro
Log Max	190	200	210
Log Reps	170/8	180/4	180/6
Yoke 75 Feet (no drops, under 15 seconds)	550	600	650
Farmer's Walk 75 Feet (no drop sub 20 sec)	225	250	275
Cement Stone	300	310	320
Cement Stone (8 reps in 60 sec)	250	265	285
Deadlift Max	450	475	500

Lifting Standards—Men

	175	231	231 Pro
Log Max	260	300	330
Log Reps	240/6	280/6	300/6
Yoke 75 Feet (no drops, under 15 seconds)	600	700	800
Farmer's Walk 75 Feet (no drop sub 20 sec)	250	275	300
Cement Stone	300	360	400
Cement Stone (8 reps in 60 sec)	250	300	360
Deadlift Max	600	650	750

	Open	Open Pro
Log Max	350	370
Log Reps	330/6	350/6
Yoke 75 Feet (no drops, under 15 seconds)	900	1000
Farmer's Walk 75 Feet (no drop sub 20 sec)	300	350
Cement Stone	425	450
Cement Stone (8 reps in 60 sec)	385	400
Deadlift Max	800	850

Final Thoughts

Success in strongman not only requires great limit strength but also event technical proficiency, explosive strength, strength endurance, and athleticism. With this book, you have the means to develop all of the above. Once you acquire a level of competency and you are chomping at the bit, competitive strongman could be the next step. So, if you want to compete, do it!

PROGRAMS

Tactical PHA Program

Thomas Hobbes described life in the state of nature as "solitary, nasty, and brutish." This description could also be used to explain Peripheral Heart Action (PHA) training. Basically, it is circuit training on steroids. Take note: This program is not for the testicular fortitude challenged!

If you have taken up training for the communal or socializing aspects, that's awesome. May you find communal glee in Spin class and booty boot camp. But this will not be the program for you.

This workout is for the hard-core garage gym dweller, for the dude who enters the commercial gym without stopping to check out the spandex parade on the cardio machine, and for every iron warrior who wants successful gains more than social status. There won't be time for selfies, setting up cameras to film, or a cheering parade at the end of the sessions.

This is about you against you.

This is a solitude journey.

Now, solitude is the state of being alone without feeling lonely. The assumption that being alone leaves you lonely is a social construct that is imposed on you. You can choose to be alone, in solitude. Solitude is a state nearly all great philosophers, mystics, athletes, and masters of their craft have embraced. As Albert Einstein said, "I live in that solitude which is painful in youth, but delicious in the years of maturity."

In the same way that you can make a choice to engage solitude, you can make a choice to follow this routine. When you drop everything and fully engage in the present moment with this training program, you'll experience solitude—and truly appreciate this constructive state of engagement with yourself.

Sound mind, body, and spirit—the Tactical PHA training program embraces and builds this sacred union.

Real Life

The benefits beyond the physical with Tactical PHA training are evident; this, however, is not a pie-in-the-sky theory. It has been used and proven in the trenches.

Initially, the Tactical PHA philosophy was guinea pigged on Taylor Lopes, a senior SWAT officer in California and one of the toughest SOBs on the planet. After a serious incident that required a foot chase of 300 yards and a physical confrontation, Lopes had the following to say: "My mental and physical preparation was on another level. I wasn't out of breath; I stayed extremely calm and handled the situation."

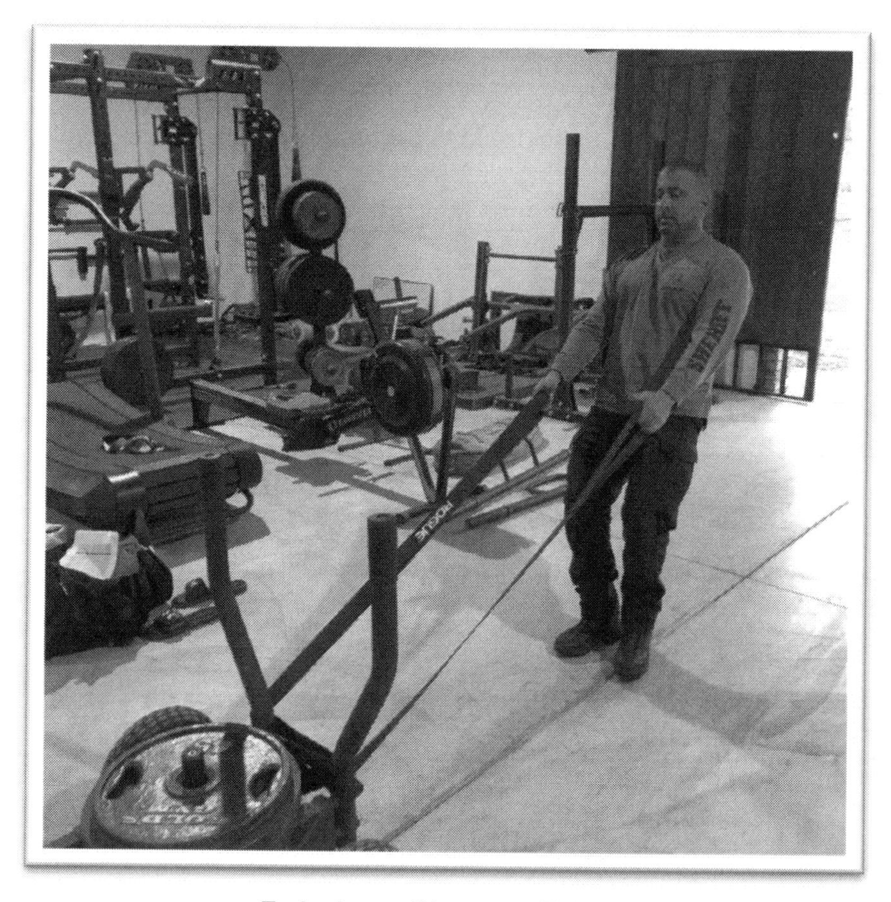

Taylor Lopes Strongman Training

This is just the tip of the iceberg. This program will not prepare you to win the Boston Marathon, but you will be ready for a multitude of real-world scenarios, from barfights to moving a new flat-screen TV into your gym crush's condo.

To benefit the most from this type of programming, an athlete should be able to minimally meet the following requirements:

- ✓ 2.0 x bodyweight squat
- ✓ 2.2 x bodyweight deadlift
- ✓ 1.2 x bodyweight pull-up
- ✓ 1.2 x bodyweight bench press
- ✓ 0.8 x bodyweight overhead press

The stronger the athlete, the more they will benefit from the Tactical PHA training program.

We suggest meeting these strength standards before engaging in this program. However, this is a recommendation, not a rule. The reason these standards are written in a strength-to-bodyweight ratio format is because that ratio has been shown numerous times to be a predictor of speed.

Logically speaking, no matter what your absolute strength is, if you can't do a pull-up, will you be able to climb over an obstruction?

We did not invent PHA training, but we tweaked it to benefit you in any kind of tactical or functional situations you could face. Understand that this is not circuit training at Planet Fitness.

This is flat-assed heavy strongman training with a synergistic blend of raw pig iron and an extreme conditioning component.

Your state will be readiness!

Circuit Training

The reason circuit training results "suck hind tit" is because most circuit training workouts are primarily done on machines sitting down. Now, when you sit down on a machine, you are no longer using your stabilizer muscles. Basically, the machine takes the workload off your stabilizing muscles. That may sound nice, but you need to put in work to work out. So, the exercises that are performed on a machine are much less metabolically demanding. This leaves you in a situation where you burn a fraction of the calories of a more demanding exercise selection.

Okay, how do you burn more calories? You turn to PHA training.

PHA History

PHA was popularized by Bob Gajda. A pioneer of the Chicago bodybuilding scene, Gajda won the Mr. Universe and Mr. America bodybuilding titles in the 1960s. PHA training focuses on keeping blood continuously circulating through the body throughout the entire workout. This is done by attacking the smaller muscles around the heart first, then moving outward.

This system is vigorous and requires continued, intense exercise for a prolonged period of time without any rest. Because of this, the mentally and physically poorly conditioned athlete should not attempt the Tactical PHA training program.

For efficient training, Gajda advocated compound movements (i.e., exercises that work multiple muscle groups at the same time). What we refer to as Tactical PHA training blends beautifully with strongman events. The goal is to "shunt" (i.e., push or pull) blood up and down the body.

This type of workout is extremely taxing on the cardiovascular system, and, unsurprisingly, the benefits are a reduction in body fat. In addition, you get an improved metabolic rate, which makes this a real Gas Station Ready type of conditioning!

With Tactical PHA training, the body parts are worked sequentially. This allows body parts to recover or, at least, to get adequate rest between each circuit. Due to the rest, your strength will be conserved, and you are able to lift heavier weights than in traditional circuit training. Even though your heart will likely beat at over 150 beats per minute throughout the entire workout, the idea is not to lower the prescribed weights.

Limit Strength

Limit strength refers to the amount of weight you can lift in one all-out effort.

Traditional circuit training removes your prospects of gaining or even maintaining limit strength.

In contrast, with our Tactical PHA training program, you are able to follow the mantra of "go heavy or go home" because you are adding more weight to the bar.

Look, you get stronger with Tactical PHA training because you're doing heavy strongman and compound movements, not the "good girl/bad girl" machine.

The bottom line is that the Tactical PHA training program accelerates fat loss but can also be used to induce muscle hypertrophy, or growth (as long as a caloric surplus is maintained throughout the program).

The Tactical PHA Training Program Explained

Perform the exercises in sequence one for the required number of reps without stopping. Repeat the sequence twice more, then move on to sequence two and perform it the same way you performed sequence one.

IMPORTANT NOTES:

✓ Take a 5 – to 10-minute break between sequence 1 and 2.

✓ Do not rest during a sequence, and do not rest between completing the same sequence for the second and third times, unless it is absolutely necessary. After all, long breaks defeat the purpose.

✓ If you need to lower the weights during week 1 beyond 10 percent, consider a different program. This program is very elitist; yes, you are certifiable "BMF" if you complete it.

Day 1/Sequence 1

Exercise	Weight or Intensity	Sets	Reps	Rest Interval	Special Notes
Dumbbell Incline Press	15-rep max	3	6-10	None	30 – to 45-degree incline angle
Squats	12-rep max	3	5-8	None	
Farmer's Walk	80%	3	50 feet	None	Use 80% of the total weight you could do for one trip for 50 feet.
Neutral-Grip Lat Pulldowns	20-rep max	3	10-15	None	
Neck Extensions	Weight you can comfortably do 40 reps with	3	20	60 sec	If you have been training neck, you can start heavier.

- Dumbbell Incline Press can be replaced with any barbell incline/decline/flat press, dumbbell flat/incline press, log incline press, push-ups (add resistance if applicable), or machine incline, decline, or flat press (machine only if working around an injury). All of these movements should be executed with the same rep/intensity scheme, unless otherwise noted.
- Squats can be replaced with front squats (rep range 4-6), Hatfield overload squats, Olympic pause squats (high bar, close stance), belt squat variations and safety squats (not holding rack), or any other specialty bar squat. All of these movements should be executed with the same rep/intensity scheme, unless otherwise noted.
- Farmer's Walk can be replaced with any carrying event, including the following, among others: yoke carry, front yoke carry, Zercher carry, duck walk, sandbag carry, Husafell stone carry, stone carry, frame carry, or any carrying event. Execute with the same intensity for the same distance, unless otherwise noted.

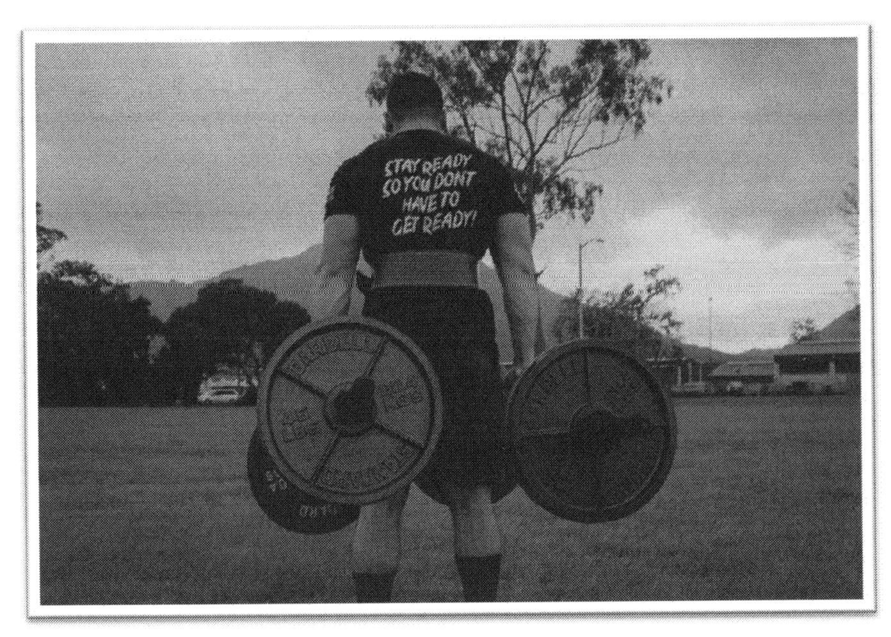

Nick DiLeo Farmer's Walk

- Neutral-Grip Lat Pulldowns: The advanced lifter can substitute neutral-grip pull-ups or any pull-up variation. Bands can be used for lat pulldowns and any pullover variation focusing on the lats. All of these movements should be executed with the same rep/intensity scheme, unless otherwise noted.
- Neck Extensions: Lie facedown on a bench with your shoulders just beyond the end. This is the starting position. Holding a weight plate firmly against the back of your head, lower your head until you feel a comfortable stretch. Under control, bring your head up briefly. Hold your head in this extended position, then lower it again. This is one rep. Substitutions with a harness, four-way neck machine, or band are all fine as long as the prescribed movement pattern is executed. All of these movements should be executed with the same rep/intensity scheme, unless otherwise noted.

Day 1/Sequence 2

Exercise	Weight or Intensity	Sets	Reps	Rest Interval	Special Notes
Lateral Step-Ups	12-rep max each leg	3	4-6 each leg	None	Athletes over 6 feet use 24-inch height, under 6 feet use 20 inches.
Lateral Raises	20-rep max	3	10-15	None	
T-Bar Prison Rows	15-rep max	3	6-8	None	
Backward Sled Drags	80%	3	60 feet	None	Use 80% of the total weight you could do for one trip for 60 feet.
Dumbbell Floor Paused Triceps Extensions	20-rep max	3	10—15	None	

- Lateral Step-Ups can be replaced with lateral lunges, sled-resisted lateral sprints (one set of 20 yards each way counts as a set), sandbag lateral lunges, sandbag lateral step-ups, 45-degree lunges, 45-degree drop lunges, or lateral box jumps/hurdle jumps. All of these movements should be executed with the same rep/intensity scheme, unless otherwise noted.
- Lateral Raises can be replaced with lateral cable raises, lean-away lateral raises, crucifix holds for 30 seconds, any rear delt movement, or upright rows. All of these movements should be executed with the same rep/intensity scheme, unless otherwise noted.
- T-Bar Prison Rows can be replaced with Yates rows, Pendlay rows, bent-over dumbbell rows, head-supported rows, log rows, one-arm dumbbell rows (5-6 reps each way is one set), Meadows rows (5-6 reps each way is one set), or seated rows. All of these movements should be executed with the same rep/intensity scheme, unless otherwise noted.
- Backward Sled Drags can be replaced with any flipping or pulling events. These include but are not limited to: truck pulls, any arm over arm pull seated or standing, Fingal's Fingers, or chain drags. All of these movements should be executed with the same rep/intensity scheme, unless otherwise noted.

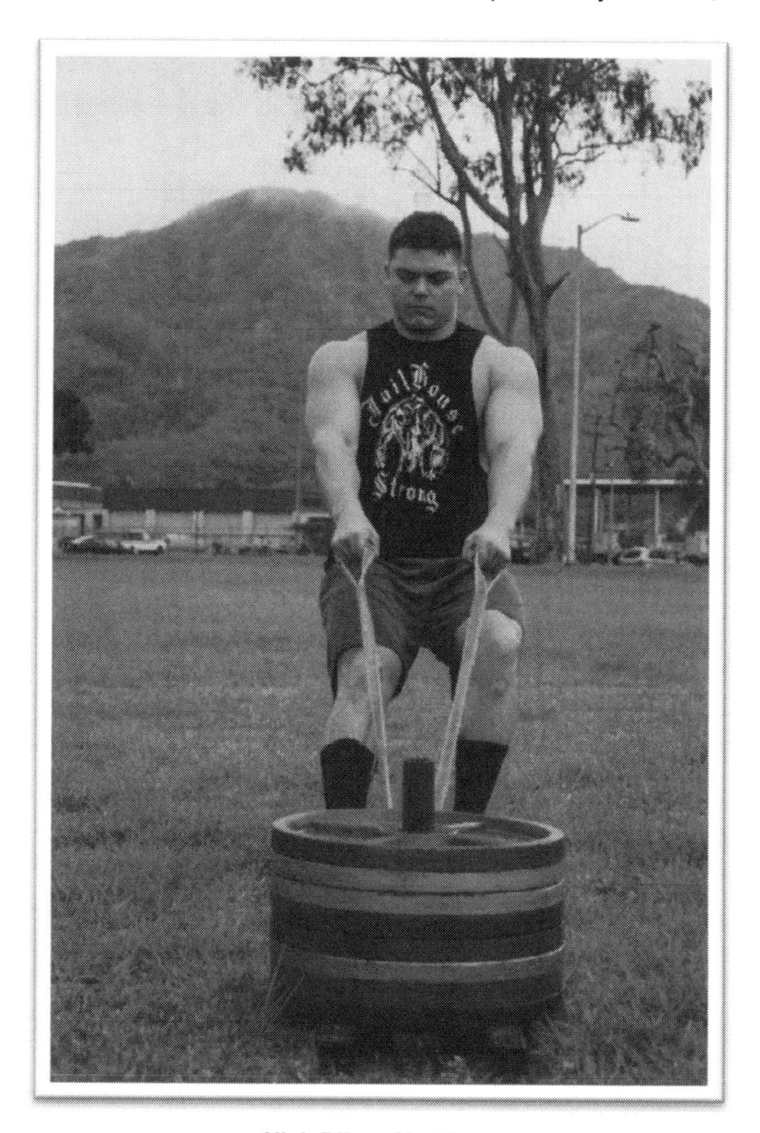

Nick DiLeo Sled Drag

- Dumbbell Floor Paused Triceps Extensions can be replaced with any barbell or dumbbell triceps extension variation. Any triceps pushdown variation is also acceptable. All of these movements should be executed with the same rep/intensity scheme, unless otherwise noted.

Day 2/Sequence 1

Exercise	Weight or Intensity	Sets	Reps	Rest Interval	Special Notes
Log Clean and Press	10-rep max	3	3-5	None	Clean and press each rep.
Sled Sprints	20% of your bodyweight	3	20 yards	None	Fast as possible
Hindu Push – Ups	Bodyweight	3	3 shy of failure	None	Form deteriora-tion is failure.
Towel Pull-Ups	8-rep max	3	3-4	None	
Neck Flexions	Weight you can comfortably do 40 reps with	3	20	60 sec	If you have been training neck, you can start heavier.

- Log Clean and Press can be replaced with the following, among others: axle clean and press, sandbag clean and press, rock clean and press, or circus dumbbell (2-3 reps each side is one set). Any barbell or dumbbell triceps extension variation is acceptable. All of these movements should be executed with the same rep/intensity scheme, unless otherwise noted.
- Sled Sprints can be replaced with any form of resisted sprints, such as parachute sprints, hill sprints, sand sprints, weighted vest sprints, jumping lunges (6 reps each leg), or sled pushes. All of these movements should be executed with the same rep/intensity scheme, unless otherwise noted.
- Hindu Push-Ups can be replaced with any bodyweight movement that targets the chest, shoulders, and triceps. All of these movements should be executed with the same rep/intensity scheme, unless otherwise noted.
- Towel Pull-Ups can be replaced with any lat pulldown or pull-up variation where a towel is used for grip. All of these movements should be executed with the same rep/intensity scheme, unless otherwise noted.
- Neck Flexions: Wear a comfortable beanie (preferably Jailhouse Strong or Gas Station Ready) or place a folded towel on your forehead to cushion the weight plate you'll be using. Lie on a bench on your back with your head hanging off the end and your feet on the floor. Place the plate on your forehead. Moving slowly, flex your head up until your chin touches your upper chest. Extend your neck backward to a comfortable stretch. Repeat for 3 sets of 20 reps. Substitutions with a harness, four-way neck machine, or band are all fine as long as the prescribed movement pattern is executed. All of these movements should be executed with the same rep/intensity scheme, unless otherwise noted.

Day 2/Sequence 2

Exercise	Weight or Intensity	Sets	Reps	Rest Interval	Special Notes
Burpees	Bodyweight	3	6-10	None	
Leg Curls	10-rep max	3	6-8	None	
EZ Curl Biceps Curls	20-rep max	3	10-12	None	Standing
Drop Lunges	10-rep max each leg	3	3-5 each leg	None	"Drop" from a 3-inch surface.
Dumbbell Pause Floor Flys	20-rep max	3	10-12	None	

- Burpees can be replaced with burpee to box jumps or up downs. All of these movements should be executed with the same rep/intensity scheme, unless otherwise noted.
- No leg curl? Band-leg curls, Nordic leg curls, or glute ham raises can be done instead. All of these movements should be executed with the same rep/intensity scheme, unless otherwise noted.
- EZ Curl Biceps Curls can be any curling variation in a strict, muscle-intention style. All of these movements should be executed with the same rep/intensity scheme, unless otherwise noted.
- Drop Lunges can be replaced with Bulgarian split squats, any step-up, or any lunge variation. All of these movements should be executed with the same rep/intensity scheme, unless otherwise noted.
- Dumbbell Pause Floor Flys can be replaced with any machine fly or dumbbell fly variation. All of these movements should be executed with the same rep/intensity scheme, unless otherwise noted.

Day 3/Sequence 1

Exercise	Weight or Intensity	Sets	Reps	Rest Interval	Special Notes
Sandbag Loads	10-rep max	3	3-5	None	Over 6 feet, use greater than 48 inches, under 6 feet, use 42 – to 48-inch surface.
Dips	15-rep max	3	6-10 reps	None	Add weight when applicable.
Yokes	75% of the total weight you could do one trip for 50 feet	3	50 feet	None	
Face Pulls	20-rep max	3	12	None	Err to the side of going light.
Side Necks	Weight you can comfortably do 20 reps with	3	10 each side	None	If you have been training neck, you can start heavier.

- Sandbag Loads can be replaced with loading events or heavy throws; examples include but are not limited to: stone loading, keg loading, stone/sandbag/keg over bar, or any other odd object load or real-world tire throw. All of these movements should be executed with the same rep/intensity scheme, unless otherwise noted.

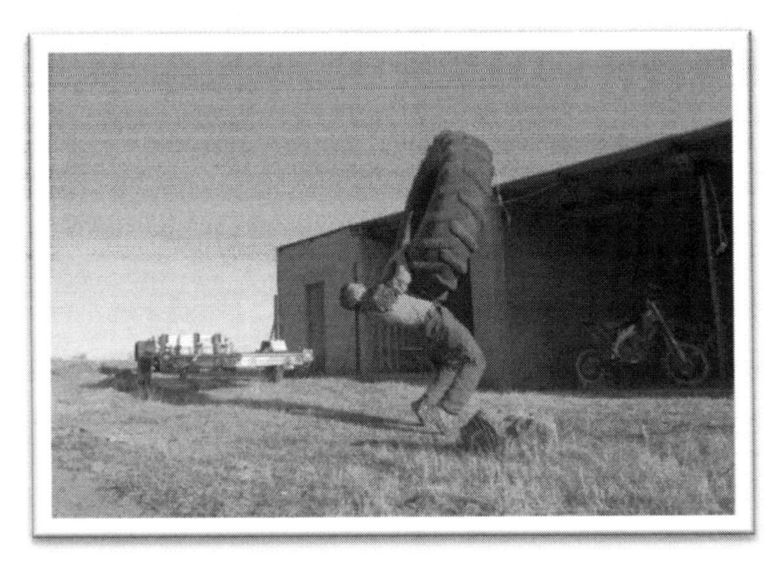

Harry Walker with a Real-World Tire Throw

- Dips: Weight can be reduced with band assistance or an assisted machine, if needed. Substitutions are push-ups or any chest press machine variation. All of these movements should be executed with the same rep/intensity scheme, unless otherwise noted.
- Yokes can be replaced with any carrying event; this can include the following exercises, among many others: chain yoke carry, Spud yoke carry, front yoke carry, Zercher carry, duck walk, sandbag carry, Husafell stone carry, farmer's walk, stone carry, frame carry, or any carrying event. Execute with the same intensity for the same distance, unless otherwise noted.

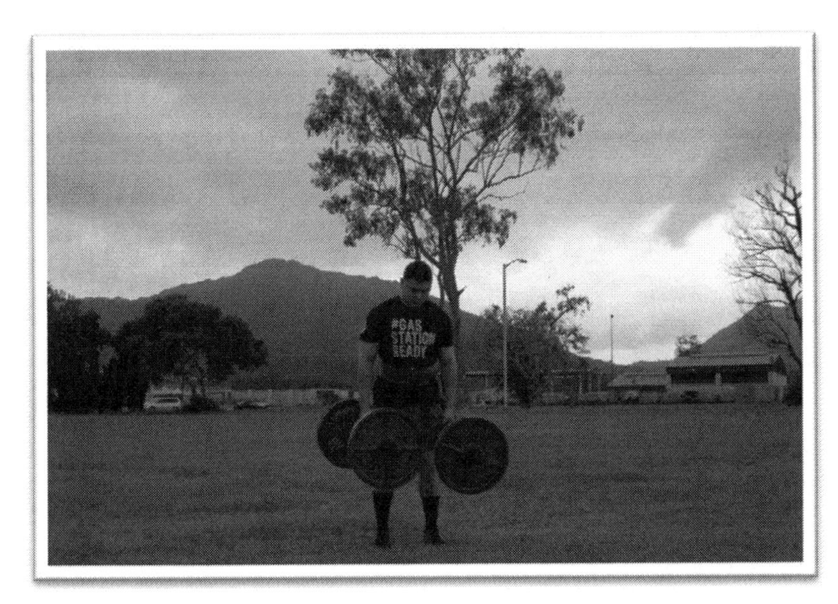

Nick DiLeo Farmer's Walk

- Face Pulls can be performed with a band, if a cable stack is not available. Execute with the same intensity for the same distance, unless otherwise noted.
- Side Necks: Place a folded towel on a weight plate. Position yourself perpendicular to a flat bench with your legs on the floor and your left forearm on the bench. Place the weight and towel on the right side of your head and hold it in place with your right hand. Move your head up to your right shoulder by laterally flexing your neck up, then laterally flex it back down again. This is one rep. Substitutions with a harness, four-way neck machine, or band are all fine as long as the prescribed movement pattern is executed. All of these movements should be executed with the same rep/intensity scheme, unless otherwise noted.

Day 3/Sequence 2

Exercise	Weight or Intensity	Sets	Reps	Rest Interval	Special Notes
Viking Press	20-rep max	3	6-10	None	
Seal Dumbbell Rows	15-rep max	3	6-10	None	
Arm over Arm Pulls	80% of the total weight you could do one trip for 50 feet	3	50 feet	None	Standing
Front Zercher Carries	75% of the total weight you could do one trip for 50 feet	3	50 feet	None	
Straight Arm Pulldowns	30-rep max	3	15-20	None	Err to the side of going light.

- Viking Press can be replaced with log clean and press, axle clean and press, sandbag clean and press, rock clean and press, circus dumbbell (2-3 reps each side is 1 set). All done in one, clean and press away style. All of these movements should be executed with the same rep/intensity scheme, unless otherwise noted.
- Seal Dumbbell Rows: Hold contraction for half a second at the top of the movement. Any chest-supported row variation can be substituted. The key is chest supported because your lower back works hard on other days of the program. All of these movements should be executed with the same rep/intensity scheme, unless otherwise noted.
- Arm over Arm Pulls: Any sort of arm over arm cable rope pull can be substituted (for more on this, see the detailed description in the Commercial Gym section). In addition, any flipping or pulling event is an acceptable substitution. All of these movements should be executed with the same rep/intensity scheme, unless otherwise noted.

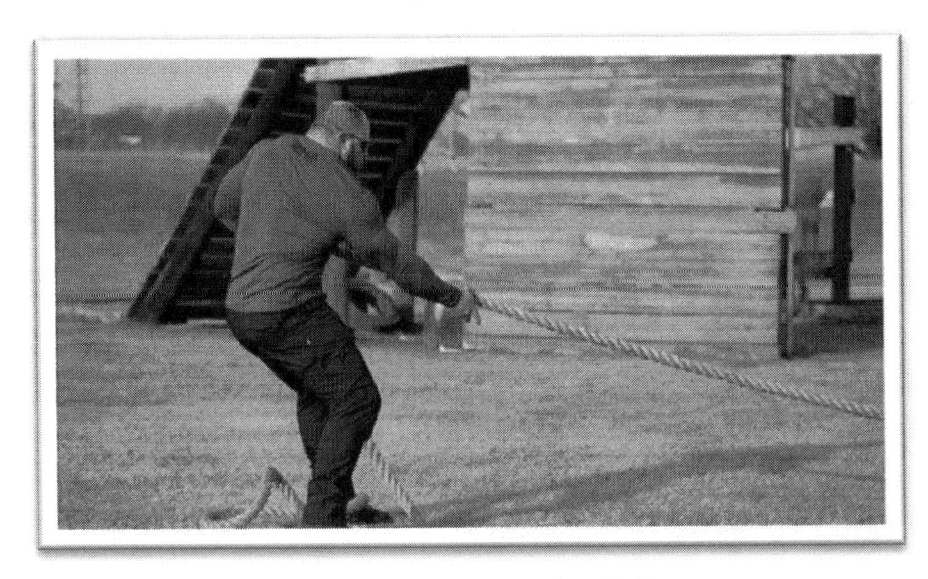

Butch Steinle Arm over Arm Pull

- Front Zercher Carries can be replaced with any carrying event. This can include exercises from the following, but far from exhaustive, list: chain yoke carry, Spud yoke carry, front yoke carry, duck walk, sandbag carry, Husafell stone carry, farmer's walk, stone carry, frame carry, or any carrying event. Execute with the same intensity for the same distance, unless otherwise noted.
- Straight Arm Pulldowns: No pulley system? Use a band or any pullover variation focusing on the lats. Execute with the same intensity for the same distance, unless otherwise noted.

Day 4

Exercise	Weight or Intensity	Sets	Reps	Rest Interval
Neutral-Grip Pull-Ups	15-rep max	3	10	60 sec
Pec Deck Rear Delt Flys	20-rep max	3	15	60 sec
Walking Lunges	Moderate	3	20 yards	60 sec
Kettlebell Swings	Moderate	3	12	60 sec
Reverse Curls	20-rep max	3	15	60 sec
Triceps Pushdowns	20-rep max	3	15	60 sec

- This day is optional. These exercises are just a sample; this day is used to target weaknesses. This day should be far easier than the other three. Execute six exercises that target your weaknesses, never approaching failure for three sets each. View it as an active recovery day.
- Other active recovery modalities: brisk walking, rucking, jump rope, elliptical, swimming, sled drags, bodyweight training, or very light lifting technique work. The idea is to keep your heart rate in the 110-135 range, in the neighborhood of 30 minutes straight. These days can be done one to three days

a week in addition to the three prescribed training sessions; remember that active recovery is 100 percent optional! ALWAYS err to the side of too little.

Variable Manipulation

We recommend sticking with the described exercises in these circuits for four to six weeks in a row. As you adapt each week, you can make the workouts more intense by referring to the bullet points.

DO NOT DO THIS WORKOUT MORE THAN SIX WEEKS IN A ROW!

The reason is that you will adapt to it quickly. Over the period of a year, you can do up to four six-week cycles.

After completing a four – to six-week run of Tactical PHA training, we recommend taking a reload/deload week.

Final Thoughts

The reason this type of training is not more popular is because personal trainers would have terrible client retention rates from the sheer pain their clients experience. No famous personal trainer or Internet personality makes money because you do PHA training. PHA training benefits only you.

Before illegal anabolic drugs hijacked many sound training principles and systems, PHA training helped construct many championship-caliber, lean, muscular physiques with functional conditioning to match.

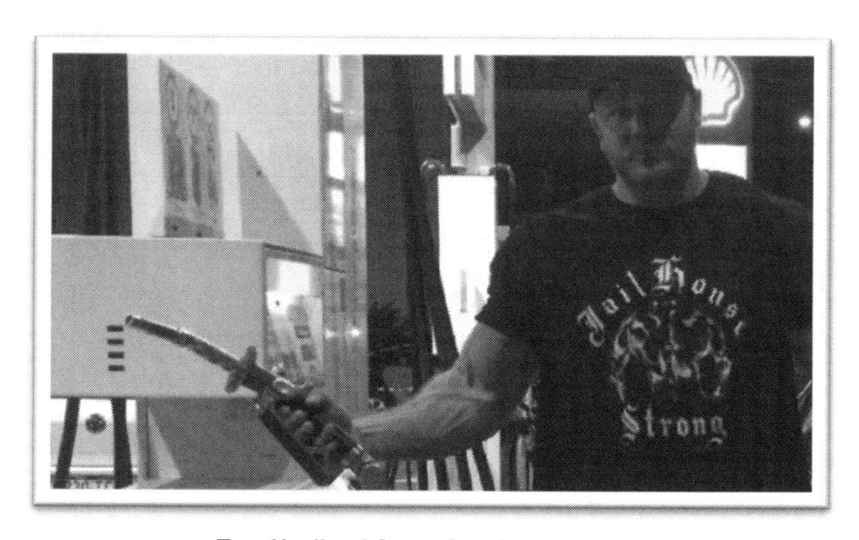

Tom Haviland Stays Gas Station Ready

Gas Station Ready Strongman Program

Size, strength, and speed are a deadly combination!

We all want to be fast and strong, but also durable enough to endure recurrent competitive seasons (be it the local softball league or farm team hockey) injury-free while staying sufficiently sharp to make it out of a dustup with the belligerent baker's dozen of *pendejos* who wait for you outside your favorite Juarez dive bar.

If you are willing to put in the work, train like an iron monk for the next eight weeks who would not miss a workout, keep a proper nutrition plan (our book, *Nutrition, Your Way* is a great place to turn for nutritional information), and avoid booze and late-night carousing, then you can expect the following:

- You will get bigger (that is, increase your lean muscle mass)
- You will get stronger through your legs, core, and upper body. You will also increase joint stability and be capable of creating higher amounts of force.
- You will become more explosive by using your muscle and strength to generate greater speed, power, and agility. You will create more force and do it faster.
- Your strength and power endurance will improve, and you will be able to display strength and power repeatedly.
- Your confidence will improve. Psychologically, you will be better prepared for social, professional, and personal challenges, and, with the improvements in your physique, you will be more confident walking into a business meeting, addressing your congregation, or taking stage on amateur night at the local exotic dancing revue.

Remember the following points:

- Upon completing the listed protocol each week, add 5 to 10 percent to the weights you used the previous week.
- When all reps in the sequences are achieved, increase the resistance.
- A week is complete as long as you hit within the rep range. Your goal should be to hit the highest end of the listed rep range during set one. So, if it says 6 to 10, go for 10 the first set. It's even better if you can match it on the subsequent sets, but remember six is a passing grade.
- For the first time you do this protocol, stay with any changes you make for the entire four to six weeks. As you advance, you can switch exercises more frequently on subsequent runs of this program.
- Strongman exercises can be swapped with something else of its "kind." So, a carrying exercise should be swapped with a carrying exercise.
- Rest for 72 to 96 hours between training days one and four and two and five. Active recovery days are not considered training days.
- If you require additional rest, lower the weight and hit the prescribed sets and reps.
- A week is complete as long as you hit the target weights and reps. If you cannot hit the target reps or weight two weeks in a row, start the program over and reduce your starting maxes by 10 percent. You can attempt the weight again the following week.
- For strongman events that must be completed in a set amount of time, rest as needed. But you must complete the prescribed sets in the allocated time. Failing to do this for two weeks in a row requires you to start over and reduce the weight by 10 percent.
- All percentages are based on *your current* maxes. We recommend starting at 95 percent of your current true one-repetition maximum (for example, a 400-pound squat would count as 380).
- Speak to your physician before starting this program.
- If you have high blood pressure, heart issues, and/or poor conditioning, avoid this program.
- Do not increase weight on core lifts. If they are easy, explode harder.
- Execute compound movement/core lifts in a movement intention/compensatory acceleration training (CAT) style by going as explosively as possible while moving from point A to point B with excellent technique.
- Execute isolation exercises by focusing specifically on the muscle you are targeting and feeling, not just moving, the weight. We refer to this as muscle intention.

- Focus on great technique. With strongman events, we would prefer that you move slightly slower with good technique (remember, this is not a contest, and you want to decrease the likelihood of injury).
- Exercise substitutions are listed below.
- Further instructions are listed under the respective days.

Week 1/Day 1

Exercise	Weight or Intensity	Sets	Reps	Rest Interval	Special Notes
Trap Bar Jumps	15% of trap bar dead-lift max	6	1	30 seconds	
Squats	85%, 70% one-rep max	5	3	120 sec	1 set at 85%, 4 sets at 70% focusing on maximum speed
Deadlifts	85%, 70% one-rep max	5	3	120 sec	1 set at 85%, 4 sets at 70% focusing on maximum speed
One-Leg Romanian Deadlifts	A weight with which you are capable of doing 6 reps each leg	3	3	60 sec	If single leg is too difficult to balance, opt for split stance.
Any strongman event you want practice on	80-90% of your maxi-mum capabilities	3	N/A	As needed	If you are capable of doing a farmer's walk with a total of 400 pounds for 50 feet, use 320-360 pounds for 50 feet here, if that is your event of choice.
Neck Extensions	Weight you can com-fortably do 40 reps with	3	20	60 sec	If you have been training neck, you can start heavier.
Landmine Anti-Rotationals	Moderately hard, a weight with which you could do 8 reps each way if going all out	2 each way	5 each way	60 sec	Very short range of motion

- Trap Bar Jumps: DO NOT INCREASE WEIGHT; if it is that easy, jump higher! If you do not have access to a trap bar or are unable to do this movement for the same sets and reps, the following are a suitable alternative: any weightless jump, backward overhead medicine ball throws, forward scoop medicine ball throws, vertical jumps with a weighted vest, real-world tire throw, high pulls (50 percent of one-rep max). All of these movements should be executed with the same rep/intensity scheme, unless otherwise noted.

- Squats can be replaced with front squats, Hatfield overload squats, Olympic pause squats (high bar close stance), belt squat variations and safety squats (not holding rack), or any other specialty bar squat. All of these movements should be executed with the same rep/intensity scheme, unless otherwise noted.
- Deadlifts can be replaced with any deadlift variation including but not limited to: Trap Bar Deadlifts, Block Deadlifts, Rack Pulls, Deficit Deadlifts, Car Deadlifts or Snatch Grip Deadlifts. All of these movements should be executed with the same rep/intensity scheme, unless otherwise noted.
- One-Leg Romanian Deadlifts can be replaced with split-stance Romanian deadlifts, snatch grip Romanian deadlifts, Nordic leg curls, or glute ham raises. All of these movements should be executed with the same rep/intensity scheme, unless otherwise noted.
- Any strongman event: We recommend doing a new one every single week. Become proficient in a multitude of events.
- Neck Extensions: Lie facedown on a bench with your shoulders just beyond the end. This is the starting position. Holding a weight plate firmly against the back of your head, lower your head until you feel a comfortable stretch. Under control, bring your head up briefly. Hold your head in this extended position, then lower it again. This is one rep. Substitutions with a harness, four-way neck machine, or band are all fine as long as the prescribed movement pattern is executed. All of these movements should be executed with the same rep/intensity scheme, unless otherwise noted.
- Landmines can be switched for any anti-rotational core movement. All of these movements should be executed with the same rep/intensity scheme, unless otherwise noted.

Week 1/Day 2

Exercise	Weight or Intensity	Sets	Reps	Rest Interval	Special Notes
Bench Press	70%	6	5	150 seconds	Last set, go for maximum reps.
Seal Rows	Maximum	6	6		Superset with bench press
Neutral-Grip Pull-Ups	Maximum	5	3	120 sec	Add resistance if applicable.
Viking Press	8-rep max	5	5		Superset with pull-ups
Dumbbell Floor Paused Triceps Extensions	15-rep max	15	5	30 sec	Cluster set
Neck Flexions	Weight you can comfortably do 40 reps with	3	20	60 sec	
Juarez Valley Push-Ups	Bodyweight	1	See notes	8-foot walk	Athletes who can bench-press 2 times bodyweight, do a Juarez Valley 20; 1.5 times bodyweight, Juarez Valley 16; 1 time or less, Juarez Valley 10.

- Bench Presses can be replaced with any barbell incline/decline/flat press, dumbbell flat/incline press, log incline press, push-ups (add resistance if applicable), or machine incline/decline/flat press (machine only if working around an injury). All of these movements should be executed with the same rep/intensity scheme, unless otherwise noted.
- Seal Rows: Hold contraction for half a second at the top of the movement. Any chest-supported row variation can be substituted. The key is chest supported because your lower back works hard on other days of the program. All of these movements should be executed with the same rep/intensity scheme, unless otherwise noted.
- Neutral Grip Pull-Ups can be substituted for a pull-up or lat pulldown variation. Add resistance or assistance, if applicable. All of these movements should be executed with the same rep/intensity scheme, unless otherwise noted.
- Viking Press can be replaced with log clean and press, axle clean and press, sandbag clean and press, rock clean and press, circus dumbbell (2-3 reps each side is 1 set). All done in a one, clean and press away style. Any barbell or dumbbell triceps extension variation is acceptable. All of these movements should be executed with the same rep/intensity scheme, unless otherwise noted.
- Dumbbell Floor Paused Triceps Extensions can be replaced with any triceps isolation exercise. All of these movements should be executed with the same rep/intensity scheme, unless otherwise noted.
- For Neck Flexions, place a folded towel on a weight plate. Position yourself perpendicular to a flat bench with your legs on the floor and your left forearm on the bench. Place the weight and towel on the right side of your head and hold it in place with your right hand. Move your head up to your right shoulder by laterally flexing your neck up, then laterally flex it back down again; this is one rep. Substitutions with a harness, four-way neck machine, or band are all fine as long as the prescribed movement pattern is executed. All of these movements should be executed with the same rep/intensity scheme, unless otherwise noted.
- The Juarez Valley Push-Up Challenge consists of ascending and descending repetitions in an alternating fashion. The repetitions are performed in descending order on all odd-numbered sets, and on even-numbered sets, reps are performed in ascending order until they finally meet in the middle.

A Juarez Valley 20 looks like this:

Set 1: 20 reps
Set 2: 1 rep
Set 3: 19 reps
Set 4: 2 reps
Set 5: 18 reps
Set 6: 3 reps
Set 7: 17 reps
Set 8: 4 reps
Set 9: 16 reps
Set 10: 5 reps
Set 11: 15 reps
Set 12: 6 reps
Set 13: 14 reps

Set 14: 7 reps
Set 15: 13 reps
Set 16: 8 reps
Set 17: 12 reps
Set 18: 9 reps
Set 19: 11 reps
Set 20: 10 reps

Between each set, walk eight feet across your "cell," keeping in the spirit that this routine evolved out of the penitentiary. Get a baseline time and strive to consistently beat it each week.

Week 1/Day 3 (see additional notes below)

- This day is to enhance recovery, not add an additional stressor that makes it more difficult to recover from your earlier workouts.

Exercise	Weight or Intensity	Sets	Reps	Rest Interval	Special Notes
Any	Active recovery	20-40 minutes	1	N/A	Keep heart rate between 120-140 for 20 to 40 minutes straight.

Active recovery modalities: brisk walking, rucking, jump rope, elliptical, swimming, sled drags, body-weight training, light agility work, low-intensity tempo runs, or very light lifting technique work. This day is 100 percent optional! **ALWAYS err to the side of too little.**

Week 1/Day 4

Exercise	Weight or Intensity	Sets	Reps	Rest Interval	Special Notes
Front Squats	60%	6	1	30 seconds	Focus on executing with maximum speed each rep.
Box Jumps (immediately after front squats)	80% of max height	6	1		Jump as high as possible and land on the box. DO NOT RAISE BOX HEIGHT.
Farmer's Walk	65% of conventional deadlift 1-rep max	6	60 feet	As needed	Rest as needed; the goal is 6 sets. Do not exceed 10 min-utes total.

Any Loading Event	75% of 1-rep max	3	3	120 sec	Focus on technique and explosive power.
Backward Sled Drags	Weight you could do 100 feet for 1 all-out set	6	60 feet	As needed	Rest as needed; the goal is 6 sets. Do not exceed 10 minutes total.
Any Carrying Event	Weight you could do 150 feet for 1 all-out set (when fresh)	4	50 feet	As needed	Rest as needed; the goal is 4 sets. Do not exceed 10 minutes total.
Side Necks	Weight you can comfortably do 40 reps with	2 each way	20	60 sec	

- Front Squats can be replaced with high-bar squats, safety squats not holding the rack, Hatfield overload squats, or pause squats. All of these movements should be executed with the same rep/intensity scheme, unless otherwise noted.
- Box Jumps can be replaced with vertical jumps or hurdle jumps. All of these movements should be executed with the same rep/intensity scheme, unless otherwise noted.
- Farmer's walks can be substituted for any carrying event. All of these movements should be executed with the same rep/intensity scheme, unless otherwise noted.
- Any Loading Event: Any loading or heavy throwing event is permissible; the objective is triple extension. All of these movements should be executed with the same rep/intensity scheme, unless otherwise noted.
- Any Carrying Event: Any carrying event is permissible. All of these movements should be executed with the same rep/intensity scheme, unless otherwise noted.
- Backward Sled Drags can be replaced with any flipping or pulling event. All of these movements should be executed with the same rep/intensity scheme, unless otherwise noted.
- Side Necks: Place a folded towel on a weight plate. Position yourself perpendicular to a flat bench with your legs on the floor and your left forearm on the bench. Place the weight and towel on the right side of your head and hold it in place with your right hand. Move your head up to your right shoulder by laterally flexing your neck up, then laterally flex it back down again; this is one rep. Substitutions with a harness, four-way neck machine, or band are all fine as long as the prescribed movement pattern is executed. All of these movements should be executed with the same rep/intensity scheme, unless otherwise noted.

Week 1/Day 5

Exercise	Weight or Intensity	Sets	Reps	Rest Interval	Special Notes
Dips	Maximum	10	10	60 seconds	Add resistance if applicable.
Towel Pull-Ups	Maximum	8	3	30 sec	Add weight if applicable.
One-Arm Dumbbell Rows	Maximum	2	20	45 sec	Knee on bench to avoid lower back fatigue
Cable Flys	Maximum	8	8	30 sec	Feel over weight
Face Pulls	Maximum	3	12	40 sec	Feel over weight
1 and ¼ Incline Dumbbell Curls	Maximum	6	6	30 sec	Feel over weight
Band-Resisted Neck Rotations	Light	2 each way	20	60 sec	Your hand can be used for manual resis-tance if no band is available.

- For all these exercises, the goal is to use the same weight across the board for all sets; if you miss a rep, lower the weight by 10 to 15 percent. The last rep of the last set should be very difficult; this will require some guessing and intuition, unlike the previous days that are exactly spelled out.
- Dips: Weight can be reduced with band assistance or an assisted machine, if needed. Substitutions are push-ups or any chest press machine variation. All of these movements should be executed with the same rep/intensity scheme, unless otherwise noted.
- Towel Pull-Ups can be replaced with any lat pulldown or pull-up variation where a towel is used for grip. All of these movements should be executed with the same rep/intensity scheme, unless other-wise noted.
- One-Arm Dumbbell Rows can be replaced with any chest supported row, inverted row, lat pulldown, or pull up. All of these movements should be executed with the same rep/intensity scheme, unless otherwise noted.
- Cable Flys can be replaced with flys; any machine fly or dumbbell fly substitution is permissible. All of these movements should be executed with the same rep/intensity scheme, unless otherwise noted.
- Face Pulls can be performed with a band, if a cable stack is not available. Execute with the same intensity for the same distance, unless otherwise noted.
- 1 and ¼ Incline Dumbbell Curls can be replaced with any barbell, dumbbell, or machine curl variation. All of these movements should be executed with the same rep/intensity scheme, unless otherwise noted.
- Band-Resisted Neck Rotations: Attach a band to a pole, power rack, or other immovable object. Place the band across your forehead slightly above eye level and step away from the immovable object so

the band pulls moderately on your head and neck. While maintaining good posture and a straight neck, rotate your head to the right so your chin is over your right shoulder, then return to the center and rotate your chin over your left shoulder. Perform 20 reps on each side, alternating from side to side for a total of 40 reps. Do this for two sets. If no band is available, self-manual resistance can be applied. All of these movements should be executed with the same rep/intensity scheme, unless otherwise noted.

Week 1/Day 6

This day is optional. These exercises are just a sample; this day is used to target weaknesses. This day should be far easier than the other three. Execute five exercises that target your weaknesses, never approaching failure for three sets each.

Exercise	Weight or Intensity	Sets	Reps	Rest Interval	Special Notes
Log Cleans	40-50% of 1-rep max	3	3	60 seconds	
Push-Ups	Bodyweight	4	Half of maximum	60 sec	
Pull-Ups	Bodyweight	4	Half of maximum	60 sec	
Triceps Pushdowns	30-rep max	3	12	60 sec	
Hammer Curls	30-rep max	3	12	60 sec	

This day can also be used for active recovery. Active recovery modalities include brisk walking, rucking, jump rope, elliptical, swimming, sled drags, bodyweight training, light agility work, low-intensity tempo runs, or very light lifting technique work. **This day is 100% optional! ALWAYS err to the side of too little.**

Remember: Regardless of what you choose to do —today, this day is to enhance recovery, not add an additional stressor that makes recovery more difficult.

It is 100 percent fine to take both days three and six off; if you are in doubt, DO! If you are feeling mentally burned out, definitely take these days off.

Week 2/Day 1

Exercise	Weight or Intensity	Sets	Reps	Rest Interval	Special Notes
Trap Bar Jumps	15% of trap bar deadlift max	6	1	30 seconds	
Squats	85%,70% of 1-rep max	6	3	120 sec	1 set at 85%, 5 sets at 70% focusing on maximum speed
Deadlifts	85%,70% of 1-rep max	6	3	120 sec	1 set at 85%, 5 sets at 70% focusing on maximum speed
One-Leg Romanian Deadlifts	Same weight as last week	3	4	60 sec	If single leg is too difficult to balance, opt for split stance.

Continue

Exercise	Weight or Intensity	Sets	Reps	Rest Interval	Special Notes
Any strongman event you want practice on	80-90% of your maximum capabilities	3	N/A	As needed	If you are capable of doing a farmer's walk with a total of 400 pounds for 50 feet, use 320-360 pounds for 50 feet here, if that is your event of choice.
Neck Extensions	Weight you can comfortably do 40 reps with	3	20	60 sec	If you have been training neck, you can start heavier.
Landmine Anti-Rotationals	Moderately hard; a weight you could do 8 reps with each way if going all-out	each 2 way	each 5 way	60 sec	Very short range of motion

- For all neck exercises, you can maintain the weight or increase up to 2.5 pounds per week, but never more than 5!

Week 2/Day 2

Exercise	Weight or Intensity	Sets	Reps	Rest Interval	Special Notes
Bench Press	70%	8	5	150 seconds	Last set, go for maximum reps.
Seal Rows	Maximum	8	8		Superset with bench press
Neutral-Grip Pull-Ups	Maximum	6	3	120 sec	Add resistance if applicable.
Viking Press	Increase 5 to 10%from last week	4	5		Superset with pull-ups
Dumbbell Floor Paused Triceps Extensions	Increase 5 to 10% from last week	12	5	30 sec	Cluster set
Neck Flexions	Weight you can comfortably do 40 reps with	3	20	60 sec	
Juarez Valley Push-Ups	Bodyweight	1	See notes	8-foot walk	The goal is to beat your baseline time, not add reps or sets.

Week 2/Day 3

Exercise	Weight or Intensity	Sets	Reps	Rest Interval	Special Notes
Any	Active recovery	20-40 minutes	1	N/A	Keep heart rate between 120-140 for 20 to 40 minutes straight.

Week 2/Day 4

Exercise	Weight or Intensity	Sets	Reps	Rest Interval	Special Notes
Front Squats	60%	6	1	30 seconds	Focus on executing with maximum speed each rep.
Box Jumps (immediately after front squat)	80% of max height	6	1		Jump as high as possible and land on the box. DO NOT RAISE BOX HEIGHT.
Farmer's Walk	70% of conventional deadlift 1-rep max	6	60 feet	N/A	Rest as needed; the goal is 6 sets. Do not exceed 10 minutes total.
Any Loading Event	75%	3	4	120 sec	Focus on technique and explosive power.
Backward Sled Drags	Increase 5 to 10% from last week	6	60 feet	N/A	Rest as needed; the goal is 6 sets. Do not exceed 10 minutes total.
Any Carrying Event	Weight you could do 120 feet for 1 all-out set (when fresh)	4	50 feet	As needed	Rest as needed; the goal is 4 sets. Do not exceed 10 minutes total.
Side Necks	Weight you can comfortably do 40 reps with	2 each way	20	60 sec	

Week 2/Day 5

Exercise	Weight or Intensity	Sets	Reps	Rest Interval	Special Notes
Dips	Maximum	10	9	60 seconds	Add resistance if applicable.
Towel Pull-Ups	Maximum	8	4	30 sec	Add weight if applicable.
One-Arm Dumbbell Rows	Maximum	2	23	45 sec	Knee on bench to avoid lower back fatigue
Cable Flys	Maximum	8	9	30 sec	Feel over weight
Face Pulls	Maximum	3	13	40 sec	Feel over weight
1 and ¼ Incline Dumbbell Curls	Maximum	6	5	30 sec	Feel over weight
Band-Resisted Neck Rotations	Light	2 each way	20	60 sec	Your hand can be used for manual resis-tance if no band is available.

- Increase weight in each exercise as you hit the required sets and reps each week.

Week 2/Day6

Exercise	Weight or Intensity	Sets	Reps	Rest Interval	Special Notes
Log Cleans	40-50% of 1-rep max	3	3	60 seconds	
Push-Ups	Bodyweight	4	Half of maximum	60 sec	
Pull-Ups	Bodyweight	4	Half of maximum	60 sec	
Triceps Pushdowns	30-rep max	3	12	60 sec	
Hammer Curls	30-rep max	3	12	60 sec	

Week 3/Day 1

Exercise	Weight or Intensity	Sets	Reps	Rest Interval	Special Notes
Trap Bar Jumps	15% of trap bar deadlift max	6	1	30 seconds	
Squats	90%,75% of 1-rep max	4	3	150 sec	1 set at 90%, 3 sets at 75% focusing on maximum speed
Deadlifts	90%,75% of 1-rep max	6	3, 2	150 sec	1 set at 90%, 5 sets at 75% focusing on maximum speed (all 5 speed sets are two reps)
One-Leg Romanian Deadlifts	Same weight as last week	3	5	60 sec	If single leg is too difficult to balance, opt for split stance.
Any strongman event you want practice on	80-90% of your maximum capabilities	3	N/A	As needed	If you are capable of doing a farmer's walk with a total of 400 pounds for 50 feet, use 320-360 pounds for 50 feet here, if that is your event of choice.
Neck Extensions	Weight you can comfortably do 40 reps with	3	20	60 sec	If you have been training neck, you can start heavier.
Landmine Anti-Rotationals	Moderately hard; a weight you could do 8 reps with each way if going all out	2 each way	5 each way	60 sec	Short range of motion

Week 3/Day 2

Exercise	Weight or Intensity	Sets	Reps	Rest Interval	Special Notes
Bench Press	70%	10	5	150 seconds	Last set, go for maximum reps.
Seal Rows	Maximum	10	10		Superset with bench press
Neutral-Grip Pull-Ups	Maximum	3	3	120 sec	Add resistance if applicable.
Viking Press	Increase 5 to 10% from last week	3	5		Superset with pull-ups
Dumbbell Floor Paused Triceps Extensions	Increase 5 pounds from last week	15	3	30 sec	Cluster set
Neck Flexions	Weight you can comfortably do 40 reps with	3	20	60 sec	
Juarez Valley Push-Ups	Bodyweight	1	See notes	8-foot walk	Athletes who can bench-press 2 times bodyweight, do a Juarez Valley 20; 1.5 times bodyweight, Juarez Valley 16; 1 time or less, Juarez Valley 10.

Week 3/Day 3

Exercise	Weight or Intensity	Sets	Reps	Rest Interval	Special Notes
Any	Active recovery	20-40 minutes	1	N/A	Keep heart rate between 120-140 for 20 to 40 minutes straight.

Week 3/Day 4

Exercise	Weight or Intensity	Sets	Reps	Rest Interval	Special Notes
Front Squats	60%	6	1	30 seconds	Focus on executing with maximum speed each rep.
Box Jumps (immediately after front squat)	80% of max height	6	1		Jump as high as possible and land on the box. DO NOT RAISE BOX HEIGHT.
Farmer's Walk	75% of conventional deadlift 1-rep max	6	60 feet	N/A	Rest as needed; the goal is 6 sets. Do not exceed 10 minutes total.
Any Loading Event	80%	3	3	120 sec	Focus on technique and explosive power.
Backward Sled Drags	Increase 5 to 10% from last week	6	60 feet	N/A	Rest as needed; the goal is 6 sets. Do not exceed 10 minutes total.
Any Carrying Event	Weight you could do 100 feet for 1 all-out set (when fresh)	4	50 feet	As needed	Rest as needed; the goal is 4 sets. Do not exceed 10 minutes total.
Side Necks	Weight you can comfortably do 40 reps with	2 each way	20	60 sec	

Week 3/Day 5

Exercise	Weight or Intensity	Sets	Reps	Rest Interval	Special Notes
Dips	Maximum	10	8	60 seconds	Add resistance if applicable.
Towel Pull-Ups	Maximum	10	3	30 sec	Add weight if applicable.
One-Arm Dumbbell Rows	Maximum	2	25	45 sec	Knee on bench to avoid lower back fatigue
Cable Flys	Maximum	6	12	30 sec	Feel over weight
Face Pulls	Maximum	3	12	40 sec	Feel over weight
1 and ¼ Incline Dumbbell Curls	Maximum	6	4	30 sec	Feel over weight
Band-Resisted Neck Rotations	Light	2 each way	20	60 sec	Your hand can be used for manual resis-tance if no band is available.

Week 3/Day6

Exercise	Weight or Intensity	Sets	Reps	Rest Interval	Special Notes
Log Cleans	40-50% of 1-rep max	3	3	60 seconds	
Push-Ups	Bodyweight	4	Half of maximum	60 sec	
Pull-Ups	Bodyweight	4	Half of maximum	60 sec	
Triceps Pushdowns	30-rep max	3	12	60 sec	
Hammer Curls	30-rep max	3	12	60 sec	

Week 4/Day 1 (Reload/Deload Week)

Exercise	Weight or Intensity	Sets	Reps	Rest Interval	Special Notes
Squats	70% of 1-rep max	3	3	120 sec	
Deadlifts	65% of 1-rep max	6	1	60 sec	
One-Leg Romanian Deadlifts	70% of Week 3	3	2	60 sec	If single leg is too difficult to balance, opt for split stance.
Any strongman event you want practice on	60-70% of your maximum capabilities	2	N/A	As needed	If you are capable of doing a farmer's walk with a total of 400 pounds for 50 feet, use 240-280 pounds for 50 feet here, if that is your event of choice.
Neck Extensions	Same as Week 3	2	12	60 sec	
Landmine Anti-Rotationals	70% of Week 3	2 each way	5 each way	60 sec	

Week 4/Day 2

Exercise	Weight or Intensity	Sets	Reps	Rest Interval	Special Notes
Bench Press	70%	2	5	150 seconds	
Seal Rows	Same as Week 3	2	6		Superset with bench press
Neutral-Grip Pull-Ups	Same as Week 3	2	3	120 sec	Add resistance if applicable.
Viking Press	Same as Week 3	2	5		Superset with pull-ups
Dumbbell Floor Paused Triceps Extensions	Same as Week 3	3	5	30 sec	
Neck Flexions	Same as Week 3	2	12	60 sec	

Week 4/Day 3

Exercise	Weight or Intensity	Sets	Reps	Rest Interval	Special Notes
Any	Active recovery	20-40 minutes	1	N/A	Keep heart rate between 120-140 for 20 to 40 minutes straight.

Week 4/Day 4

Exercise	Weight or Intensity	Sets	Reps	Rest Interval	Special Notes
Front Squats	60%	6	1	30 seconds	Focus on executing with maximum speed each rep.
Box Jumps (immediately after front squat)	80% of max height	6	1		Jump as high as possible and land on the box. DO NOT RAISE BOX HEIGHT.
Farmer's Walk	65% of conventional deadlift 1 – rep max	2	60 feet	As needed	
Any Loading Event	55%	2	3	120 sec	Focus on technique and explosive power.
Backward Sled Drags	Same as Week 3	2	60 feet	N/A	
Side Necks	Weight you can comfortably do 40 reps with	2 each way	20	60 sec	

Week 4/Day 5

Exercise	Weight or Intensity	Sets	Reps	Rest Interval	Special Notes
Dips	Same as Week 3	2	10	60 seconds	Add resistance if applicable.
Towel Pull-Ups	Same as Week 3	3	3	30 sec	Add weight if applicable.
One-Arm Dumbbell Rows	Same as Week 3	2	8	45 sec	Knee on bench to avoid lower back fatigue
Cable Flys	Same as Week 3	2	8	30 sec	Feel over weight
Face Pulls	Same as Week 3	3	12	40 sec	Feel over weight
1 and ¼ Incline Dumbbell Curls	Same as Week 3	2	6	30 sec	Feel over weight
Band-Resisted Neck Rotations	Same as Week 3	1	12	60 sec	Your hand can be used for manual resis-tance if no band is available.

Week 4/Day6

- ***OFF—COMPLETE REST THIS DAY!***

Congratulations! You have successfully completed the first training block! Now, on to block two.

Week 5/Day 1

Exercise	Weight or Intensity	Sets	Reps	Rest Interval	Special Notes
Trap Bar Jumps	15% of trap bar deadlift max	6	1	30 seconds	
Squats	95%,77.5% of 1-rep max	4	2,3	180 sec	1 set of 2 reps at 95%, 3 sets of 3 reps at 77.5% focusing on maxi-mum speed
Deadlifts	95%,80% of 1-rep max	4	2	180 sec	1 set at 95%, 3 sets at 80% focusing on maximum speed
Glute Ham Raises	Maximum	3	3	60 sec	Add resistance if applicable.

Any strongman event you want practice on	90-100% of your maximum capabilities	3	N/A	As needed	If you are capable of doing a farmer's walk with a total of 400 pounds for 50 feet, use 360-400 pounds for 50 feet here, if that is your event of choice.
Neck Extensions	Weight you can comfortably do 40 reps with	3	20	60 sec	If you have been training neck, you can start heavier.
Palloff Press	Moderately hard, a weight you could do 8 reps with each way if going all out	2 each way	5 each way	60 sec	Band or cable

- Glute Ham Raises can be replaced with one-leg RDLs, leg curls, Nordic leg curls, TRX leg curls, or snatch grip RDLs. All of these movements should be executed with the same rep/intensity scheme, unless otherwise noted.
- Palloff Press can be replaced with any anti-rotational core movement. All of these movements should be executed with the same rep/intensity scheme, unless otherwise noted.

Week 5/Day 2

Exercise	Weight or Intensity	Sets	Reps	Rest Interval	Special Notes
Bench Press	80%, 70%	2	Rest pause	150 seconds	Stop 1 rep shy of failure.
Seal Rows	Maximum	5	5	120 sec	
Neutral-Grip Pull-Ups	Maximum	3	5	120 sec	Add resistance if applicable.
Viking Press	80%, 70%	2	Rest pause		Stop 1 rep shy of failure.
Decline Dumbbell 1 and ¼ Triceps Extensions	Maximum	8	4	90 sec	Good stretch
Neck Flexions	Weight you can comfortably do 40 reps with	3	20	60 sec	
Juarez Valley Push-Ups	Bodyweight	1	See notes	8-foot walk	Athletes who can bench-press 2 times bodyweight, do a Juarez Valley 20; 1.5 times bodyweight, Juarez Valley 16; 1 time or less, Juarez Valley 10.

- Bench Press rest pause and Viking press rest pause: "Rest pause" means execute a set at the prescribed weight doing as many reps as possible but stopping 1 rep shy of failure, rest 20 seconds, go to 1 shy of failure again, then do the same thing again, so 3 total sets to 1 rep shy of failure is 1 rest-pause set. For example, if someone has a bench press of 300 pounds, they would use 80%, or 240 pounds, and the rep scheme may be something like 7 reps, 3 reps, and 1 rep. After which, they would wait 150 seconds before doing their next set with 70%, or 210 pounds, for another rest-pause set.
- Decline Dumbbell 1 and ¼ Triceps Extensions: Do a ¼ rep at the bottom of each triceps extension, then return to the bottom and do a full rep. These can be replaced with any triceps isolation movement done in this style. All of these movements should be executed with the same rep/intensity scheme, unless otherwise noted.

Week 5/Day 3

Exercise	Weight or Intensity	Sets	Reps	Rest Interval	Special Notes
Any	Active recovery	20-40 minutes	1	N/A	Keep heart rate between 120-140 for 20 to 40 minutes straight.

Week 5/Day 4

Exercise	Weight or Intensity	Sets	Reps	Rest Interval	Special Notes
Front Squats	60%	6	1	30 seconds	Focus on executing with maximum speed each rep.
Burpee to Box Jumps (immediately after front squat)	80% of max height	6	1		Jump as high as possible and land on the box. DO NOT RAISE BOX HEIGHT.
Farmer's Walk	80% of conventional deadlift 1-rep max	6	60 feet	N/A	Rest as needed; the goal is 6 sets. Do not exceed 10 minutes total.
Any Loading Event	80%	3	5	120 sec	Focus on technique and explosive power.
Backward Sled Drags	Increase 5 to 10% from Week 3	6	60 feet	N/A	Rest as needed; the goal is 6 sets. Do not exceed 10 minutes total.
Any Carrying Event	Weight you could do 75 feet for 1 all-out set (when fresh)	2	50 feet	As needed	
Side Necks	Weight you can comfortably do 40 reps with	2 each way	20	60 sec	

- Burpee to Box Jumps can be replaced with a vertical jump, box jump, hurdle jump, or knees to feet jump. All of these movements should be executed with the same rep/intensity scheme, unless otherwise noted.

Week 5/Day 5

Exercise	Weight or Intensity	Sets	Reps	Rest Interval	Special Notes
Dips	Maximum	10	7	60 seconds	Add resistance if applicable.
Towel Pull-Ups	Maximum	10	4	30 sec	Add weight if applicable.
Seated Cable Wide Neutral-Grip Rows	15-rep max	15	4	20 sec	Clusters
Dumbbell Pause Floor Flys	Maximum	5	15	30 sec	Feel over weight
Face Pulls	Maximum	3	12	40 sec	Feel over weight
Gironda Perfect Curls	Maximum	3	8	30 sec	Feel over weight
Band-Resisted Neck Rotations	Light	2 each way	20	60 sec	Your hand can be used for manual resistance if no band is available.

- Seated Cable Wide Neutral-Grip Rows can be replaced with any seated or chest-supported rowing movement. All of these movements should be executed with the same rep/intensity scheme, unless otherwise noted.
- Dumbbell Pause Floor Flys can be replaced with any cable, dumbbell, or band fly variation. All of these movements should be executed with the same rep/intensity scheme, unless otherwise noted.
- Gironda Perfect Curls can be replaced with any machine, barbell, or dumbbell curl variation. All of these movements should be executed with the same rep/intensity scheme, unless otherwise noted.

Week 5/Day6

Exercise	Weight or Intensity	Sets	Reps	Rest Interval	Special Notes
Log Cleans	40-50% of 1-rep max	3	3	60 seconds	
Push-Ups	Bodyweight	4	Half of maximum	60 sec	
Pull-Ups	Bodyweight	4	Half of maximum	60 sec	
Triceps Pushdowns	30-rep max	3	12	60 sec	
Hammer Curls	30-rep max	3	12	60 sec	

Day 6 in this program is always optional. This day can also be used as an active recovery day. This is a lower-intensity day used to target weaknesses. These exercises are examples, not prescriptions like the other 5 days.

Week 6/Day 1

Exercise	Weight or Intensity	Sets	Reps	Rest Interval	Special Notes
Trap Bar Jumps	15% of trap bar deadlift max	6	1	30 seconds	
Squats	97.5%,80% of 1-rep max	4	2,3	180 sec	1 set of 2 reps at 97.5%, 3 sets of 3 reps at 80% focusing on maximum speed
Deadlifts	102.5%,80% of 1-rep max	4	1,2	180 sec	1 set of 1 rep at 102.5%, 3 sets of 2 reps at 80% focusing on maximum speed
Glute Ham Raises	Maximum	3	4	60 sec	Add resistance if applicable.
Any strongman event you want practice on	95—100% of your maximum capabilities	2	N/A	As needed	If you are capable of doing a farmer's walk with a total of 400 pounds for 50 feet, use 380-400 pounds for 50 feet here, if that is your event of choice.
Neck Extensions	Weight you can comfortably do 40 reps with	2 each way	20	60 sec	If you have been training neck, you can start heavier.
Palloff Press	Moderately hard, a weight you could do 8 reps with each way if going all out	2 each way	5 each way	60 sec	Band or cable

Week 6/Day 2

Exercise	Weight or Intensity	Sets	Reps	Rest Interval	Special Notes
Bench Press	85%, 72.5%	2	Rest pause	150 seconds	Stop 1 rep shy of failure.
Seal Rows	Maximum	5	5	120 sec	
Neutral-Grip Pull-Ups	Maximum	4	5	120 sec	Add resistance if applicable.
Viking Press	80%, 70%	2	Rest pause		Stop 1 rep shy of failure.
Decline Dumbbell 1 and ¼ Triceps Extensions	Maximum	4	9	90 sec	Good stretch
Neck Flexions	Weight you can comfortably do 40 reps with	3	20	60 sec	
Juarez Valley Push-Ups	Bodyweight	1	See notes	8-foot walk	Athletes who can bench-press 2 times bodyweight, do a Juarez Valley 20; 1.5 times bodyweight, Juarez Valley 16; 1 time or less, Juarez Valley 10.

Week 6/Day 3

Exercise	Weight or Intensity	Sets	Reps	Rest Interval	Special Notes
Any	Active recovery	20-40 minutes	1	N/A	Keep heart rate between 120-140 for 20 to 40 minutes straight.

Week 6/Day 4

Exercise	Weight or Intensity	Sets	Reps	Rest Interval	Special Notes
Front Squats	60%	6	1	30 seconds	Focus on executing with maximum speed each rep.
Burpee to Box Jumps (immediately after front squat)	80% of max height	6	1		Jump as high as possible and land on the box. DO NOT RAISE BOX HEIGHT.
Farmer's Walk	85% of conventional deadlift 1-rep max	5	50 feet	N/A	Rest as needed; the goal is 5 sets. Do not exceed 10 minutes total.
Any Loading Event	85%	3	3	120 sec	Focus on technique and explosive power.
Backward Sled Drags	Increase 5 to 10% from last week	6	60 feet	N/A	Rest as needed; the goal is 6 sets. Do not exceed 10 minutes total.
Any Carrying Event	Weight you could do 65 feet for 1 all-out set	2	50 feet	As needed	
Side Necks	Weight you can comfortably do 40 reps with	2 each way	20	60 sec	

Week 6/Day 5

Exercise	Weight or Intensity	Sets	Reps	Rest Interval	Special Notes
Dips	Maximum	10	6	60 seconds	Add resistance if applicable.
Towel Pull-Ups	Maximum	10	5	30 sec	Add weight if applicable.
Seated Cable Wide Neutral-Grip Rows	15-rep max	15	5	20 sec	Clusters
Dumbbell Pause Floor Flys	Maximum	5	13	30 sec	Feel over weight
Face Pulls	Maximum	3	12	40 sec	Feel over weight
Gironda Perfect Curls	Maximum	3	9	30 sec	Feel over weight
Band-Resisted Neck Rotations	Light	2 each way	20	60 sec	Your hand can be used for manual resistance if no band is available.

Week 6/Day 6

Exercise	Weight or Intensity	Sets	Reps	Rest Interval	Special Notes
Log Cleans	40-50% of 1-rep max	3	3	60 seconds	
Push-Ups	Bodyweight	4	Half of maximum	60 sec	
Pull-Ups	Bodyweight	4	Half of maximum	60 sec	
Triceps Pushdowns	30-rep max	3	12	60 sec	
Hammer Curls	30-rep max	3	12	60 sec	

Day 6 in this program is always optional. This day can also be used as an active recovery day. This is a lower-intensity day used to target weaknesses. These exercises are examples, not prescriptions like the other 5 days.

Week 7/Day 1

Exercise	Weight or Intensity	Sets	Reps	Rest Interval	Special Notes
Trap Bar Jumps	15% of trap bar deadlift max	6	1	30 seconds	
Squats	102.5%,82% of 1-rep max	4	1,3	180 sec	1 set of 1 rep at 102.5%, 3 sets of 3 reps at 82% focusing on maximum speed
Deadlifts	97%,75% of 1-rep max	6	2	180 sec	1 set of 2 reps at 97%, 5 sets of 2 reps at 75% focusing on maximum speed
Glute Ham Raises	Maximum	3	4	60 sec	Add resistance if applicable.
Any strongman event you want practice on	Heavy as possible	2	N/A	As needed	Let it rip.
Neck Extensions	Weight you can comfortably do 40 reps with	2 each way	20	60 sec	If you have been training neck, you can start heavier.
Palloff Press	Moderately hard, a weight you could do 8 reps with each way if going all out	2 each way	5 each way	60 sec	Band or cable

Week 7/Day 2

Exercise	Weight or Intensity	Sets	Reps	Rest Interval	Special Notes
Bench Press	88%, 70%	2	Rest pause	150 seconds	Stop 1 rep shy of failure.
Seal Rows	Maximum	5	6	120 sec	Add resistance if applicable.
Neutral-Grip Pull-Ups	Maximum	4	6	120 sec	
Viking Press	Attempt 1-rep max	3	1	As needed	Take 3 attempts to find new 1-rep max.
Decline Dumbbell 1 and ¼ Triceps Extensions	Maximum	4	10	90 sec	Good stretch
Neck Flexions	Weight you can comfortably do 40 reps with	3	20	60 sec	
Juarez Valley Push-Ups	Bodyweight	1	See notes	8-foot walk	Athletes who can bench-press 2 times bodyweight, do a Juarez Valley 20; 1.5 times bodyweight, Juarez Valley 16; 1 time or less, Juarez Valley 10.

Week 7/Day 3

Exercise	Weight or Intensity	Sets	Reps	Rest Interval	Special Notes
Any	Active recovery	20-40 minutes	1	N/A	Keep heart rate between 120-140 for 20 to 40 minutes straight.

Week 7/Day 4

Exercise	Weight or Intensity	Sets	Reps	Rest Interval	Special Notes
Front Squats	60%	6	1	30 seconds	Focus on executing with maximum speed each rep.
Burpee to Box Jumps (immediately after front squat)	80% of max height	6	1		Jump as high as possible and land on the box. DO NOT RAISE BOX HEIGHT.
Farmer's Walk	90% of conventional deadlift 1-rep max	4	40 feet	N/A	Rest as needed; the goal is 5 sets. Do not exceed 10 minutes total.
Any Loading Event	90%	3	3	120 sec	Focus on technique and explosive power.
Backward Sled Drags	Increase 5 to 10% from last week	6	60 feet	N/A	Rest as needed; the goal is 6 sets. Do not exceed 10 minutes total.
Any Carrying Event	Heavy as possible	2	50 feet	As needed	
Side Necks	Weight you can comfortably do 40 reps with	2 each way	20	60 sec	

Week 7/Day 5

Exercise	Weight or Intensity	Sets	Reps	Rest Interval	Special Notes
Dips	Maximum	10	5	60 seconds	Add resistance if applicable.
Towel Pull-Ups	Maximum	10	3	30 sec	Add weight if applicable.
Seated Cable Wide Neutral-Grip Rows	15-rep max	15	6	20 sec	Clusters
Dumbbell Pause Floor Flys	Maximum	5	15	30 sec	Feel over weight
Face Pulls	Maximum	3	12	40 sec	Feel over weight
Gironda Perfect Curls	Maximum	3	9	30 sec	Feel over weight
Band-Resisted Neck Rotations	Light	2 each way	20	60 sec	Your hand can be used for manual resistance if no band is available.

Week 7/Day 6

Exercise	Weight or Intensity	Sets	Reps	Rest Interval	Special Notes
Log Cleans	40-50% of 1-rep max	3	3	60 seconds	
Push-Ups	Bodyweight	4	Half of maximum	60 sec	
Pull-Ups	Bodyweight	4	Half of maximum	60 sec	
Triceps Pushdowns	30-rep max	3	12	60 sec	
Hammer Curls	30-rep max	3	12	60 sec	

Day 6 in this program is always optional. This day can also be used as an active recovery day.

This is a lower-intensity day used to target weaknesses. These exercises are examples, not prescriptions like the other 5 days.

Week 8

For Week 8, repeat the Week 4 Deload/Reload week.

Week 9

Congratulations! You are now bigger, faster, and stronger! If you need a week off from training, take it. You can also use this week to test maxes on any lift or strongman events. We recommend not using this program more than three times in a year and taking a minimum of a six-week break before attempting it again.

Final Thoughts

When you follow the Tactical PHA training program and/or the Gas Station Ready strongman program to completion, you have grown stronger both mentally and physically. If you prefer to design your own program, you also now have the knowledge to do so.

No matter what you do—THANK YOU! Thank you for supporting us by purchasing this book.

Because of people like you, we get to pursue our passion daily.

Please let us know how you do with these programs by tagging us on Instagram @Jailhousestrong.

BONUS MATERIAL

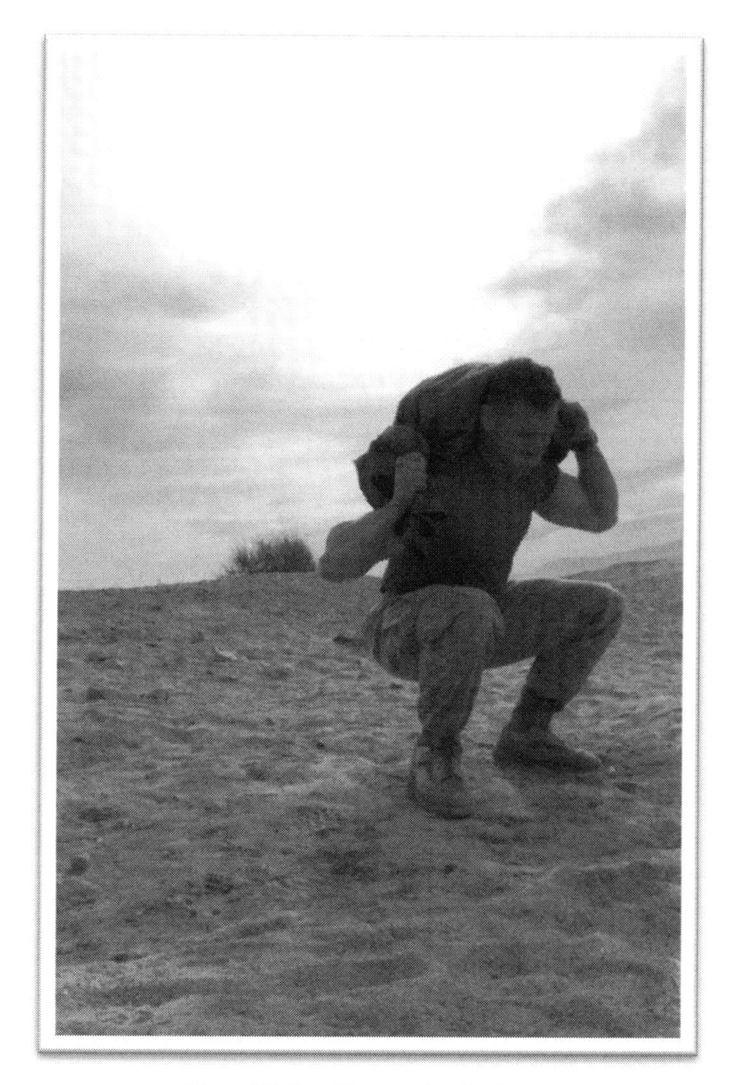

Harry Walker No Bar, No Problem

Strongman: The Science

In suburban strip mall sports performance facilities, pseudo–strength coaches hoodwink well-meaning parents into believing that "speed ladders" are their child's messianic savior for achieving increased speed and agility.

Now, to make sure that we are on the same page, increased speed means that you cover more distance in less time. Agility is the ability to rapidly change directions.

With a speed ladder drill, your center of mass doesn't move (i.e., you haven't changed directions)! So you haven't improved your agility. All you have done is move your legs without falling over. And you sure as hell haven't covered more ground faster. So you have not achieved more speed. So why is this drill implemented?

Bottom line, flash sells.

And when flash doesn't require much intestinal fortitude (like a ladder drill), it sells that much better. There is nothing wrong with a speed ladder as part of a warm-up or activation. There is something wrong if you are using it for building speed and agility.

Strongman training is not a feature of most mainstream strength, conditioning, and fitness programs because it's excruciating and it's not a major money maker for large equipment manufacturers. However, there is no type of strength training more functional than strongman training, and we have the results along with the scientific studies to prove it. So let's take a look at what science says and what that means to you.

Winwood, P. W., Cronin, J. B., Posthumus, L. R., Finlayson, S. J., Gill, N. D., and Keogh, J. W. (2015). Strongman vs. Traditional Resistance Training Effects on Muscular Function and Performance. *Journal of Strength and Conditioning Research*, 29(2), 429–439. doi: 10.1519/jsc.0000000000000629

This study compared seven weeks of strongman training with seven weeks of traditional resistance training and examined body composition, strength, power, and speed measures.

The traditional group's training routine is listed in the table below:

Exercise	Sets	Reps	Load % of 1-Rep Max	Rest Interval
Clean and Jerks	3	5	70%	3 min
Deadlifts	3	5	80%	3 min
Military Press	3	6	80%	3 min
Back Squats	3	5	85%	3 min
1-Arm Rows	2	8	35% of bent row	3 min

The strongman group's routine is listed in the table below:

Exercise	Sets	Reps	Load % of 1-Rep Max	Rest Interval
Log Lifts	3	5	70%	3 min
Farmer's Walk	3	28 meters	80% of 1-rep max deadlift	3 min
Axle Press	3	6	80% of 1-rep max military press	3 min
Heavy Sled Pulls	3	25 meters	85% of 1-rep max back squat	3 min
Arm over Arm Prowler Pulls	2	8 each arm	100% of bent row	3 min

The subjects in the study were 30 rugby players with advanced weight training experience.

Subjects were assigned to the traditional group or the strongman group. Each group was required to perform their respective routines twice weekly, and researchers selected exercises with similar biomechanics and an equivalent intensity of load.

Subjects were assessed for body composition, strength, power, speed, and change of direction speed. All performance markers in both groups improved. No significant differences between groups in functional performance were observed after seven weeks of following their respective routines.

Breaking it down further, the strongman group compared to the traditional group had greater increases in muscle mass, acceleration performance, and the bent-over row. The traditional group had greater increases in squat and deadlift performance, horizontal jump, and change of direction ability.

Researchers confirmed the efficacy of strongman training and believe short-term strongman programs are as effective as traditional lifting programs for improving body composition, strength, and performance.

Takeaway Point

Strongman training is the ultimate hybrid of powerlifting, Olympic lifting, and bodybuilding. It truly bridges the gap between the weight room and the field of play! Programs rarely prescribe strongman only training. Instead of operating within a myopic view, embrace the synergy of combining strongman training with traditional lifting!

Hindle, B., Winwood, P., Lorimer, A., and Keogh, J. (n.d.).

36th Conference of the International Society of Biomechanics in Sports, Auckland, New Zealand, September 10-14, 2018.

The sport of strongman has rapidly increased in popularity over the past 10 years. Strongman events are termed a functional form of resistance training. This is because strongman events involve an athlete lifting, carrying, pulling, or pushing awkward and heavy objects for a number of repetitions or for a set distance. In contrast to traditional weightlifting modalities, which typically require a weight to be lifted vertically and use bilateral load distribution, strongman events test athletes in multiple planes, involving both bilateral and unilateral loading.

This review was a literature search that was conducted to identify studies comparing biomechanical parameters of strongman events and technically similar traditional weight training exercises. Many similarities were identified. Interestingly, it was found that the farmer's lift may reduce the stress placed on the lumbar spine when compared to the deadlift performed under identical loading conditions.

Furthermore, heavy sled pulls were shown to better develop anterior force production than the back squat. In addition, the log lift can be used to better develop forceful hip extension during a triple extension movement than the clean and jerk.

The review concluded that because of biomechanical similarities between strongman events and traditional weight training lifts, strongman events can be used as an alternative to traditional lifting to develop size, strength, and power!

Takeaway Point

There is nothing more functional than picking up heavy weight off the ground and moving with it. But this review further shows that strongman events are often safer than barbell lifts and can produce superior anterior force and develop more powerful hip extension than Olympic lifts!

Hindle, B. R., Lorimer, A., Winwood, P., and Keogh, J. W. L. (2019). The Biomechanics and Applications of Strongman Exercises: A Systematic Review. *Sports Medicine* – Open, 5(1). doi: 10.1186/s40798-019-0222-z

The objective of this review of 11 studies was to establish the understanding biomechanically of strongman movements, specifically within the following scope:

(1) Improve athlete performance by providing athletes and coaches with a greater understanding of the key biomechanical factors of performance of these movements
(2) Provide biomechanical evidence that supports the transfer of training strongman movements to the strength and conditioning/rehab programs of traditional and tactical athletes along with other labor-intensive labor professions
(3) Ascertain the holes in contemporary knowledge of the biomechanics of strongman movements

Strongman movements which had a biomechanical assessment in at least one of the 11 studies included the:

- atlas stone lift
- farmer's walk
- heavy sled/vehicle pull
- log lift
- keg walk
- suitcase carry
- tire flip
- yoke walk

These eight strongman movements could be branded into three exercise types: carrying/walking, pulling, and static lifting. The comparative analyses within each of the studies are broken down to three primary areas: contrasts built on the performance result of the movement, within movement comparisons (between phase), and between exercise evaluations.

The key findings to the study were:

- Athletes with a superior overall performance outcome in the farmer's walk and heavy sled pull can be biomechanically described by a larger stride length and greater stride frequency and reduced ground contact time, while superior performance in the tire flip can be biomechanically described by a decreased second pull phase time.
- Biomechanical likenesses were recognized and shown with the strongman farmer's walk and yoke walk, and loaded backpack carriage (exciting implications for tactical athletes constantly under load); the strongman vehicle pull, and heavy sled pull and sub-body mass sled pull; and the strongman atlas stone lift, log lift, and tire flip, and numerous phases of the clean and jerk, squat, and deadlift.
- The current literature established a lack of basic measurable biomechanical data of the yoke walk, unilateral load carriage, vehicle pull, atlas stone lift, and tire flip, and biomechanical performance determinants of the log lift.

Takeaway Point

For success in competitive strongman, athletes can use this information to better improve performance. However, remember that unless you are a competitive strongman with years of experience, start off slowly and methodically. Strongman training further offers a great modality for tactical athletes to train.

Zemke, B., and Wright, G. (2011). The Use of Strongman Type Implements and Training to Increase Sport Performance in Collegiate Athletes. *Strength and Conditioning Journal*, 33(4), 1–7. doi: 10.1519/ssc.0b013e3182221f96

This article from the *Strength and Conditioning Journal* examines the use of strongman events in collegiate strength and conditioning settings. The article cites 25 relevant studies along with looking at the authors' practical experience.

Various strongman movements are similar to movements in sports. Training with strongman implements has the greatest transfer to contact sports, such as wrestling, rugby, football, and hockey. In particular, tire flips and loading atlas stones have great similarities with blocking and tackling in football. Furthermore, the simultaneous extension of the ankle, knee, and hip (triple extension) is a movement that, when executed explosively, is essential to athletic prowess.

A vast array of strongman exercises, including loading atlas stones, tire flips, and log clean and jerks, not only include powerful triple extension but emphasize core stability. Additionally, coaches who think outside the box can have athletes throw kegs and tires for explosive torso training in various dimensions.

Carrying movements, like keg or sandbag carries and farmer's walk, train the isometric holding strength along with the specific endurance needed in sports like wrestling. Grip strength and "bear hug" strength (we call this constriction strength) decrease notably over the course of a wrestling match. In regard to this, training with strongman movements that develop these types of strength becomes increasingly beneficial the longer a wrestling match continues.

In pressing exercises, like the log, the handles are in a neutral-grip position. This better mimics hand positions generally used in sports (this is in contrast to a pronated grip with a traditional barbell). Of course, coaches can manipulate these events to be performed for a sport-specific duration or number of repetitions.

Including strength and balance during lateral movement is important in many sports. To enhance lateral movement, look no further than strongman movements. Orthodox strength training exercises for lateral movement are frequently limited to things like lateral lunges, which are difficult to perform with heavy weight. With strongman training, the possibilities are endless.

Lateral movements can be done with a heavy sandbag on one or both shoulders, or even held overhead, farmer's walk implements, kegs, or a bar held in front of the body in the Zercher position. In conclusion, using strongman implements to train lateral movement expands the number of movements at the coach's/athlete's disposal. It also increases the number of different stresses placed on the body and the overall stress because heavier loads are used.

One of the areas that strongman training can have its biggest impact is in conditioning. Using strongman implements will have the greatest effect on the phosphagen and glycolytic energy systems. Explosive repeated movements that require high levels of power are required by many sports, such as football. Extensive training for a sport can be accomplished using exercises that develop the prime movers of the movements used in the specific sport, matching the amplitude and direction of the movement, joint angles used, the rate and timing of force production, and the dominant energy systems used.

Takeaway Point

Strongman offers a fun, novel, and *very effective* training stimulus, when properly incorporated into a training program. Strongman implements offer unique challenges to athletes that cannot be duplicated in the weight room. Furthermore, athletes enjoy the variety in their routines that strongman training offers. Outside of competitive strongman, strongman event training has the biggest carryover to contact sport and tactical athletes.

McGill, S. (2010). Core Training: Evidence Translating to Better Performance and Injury Prevention. *Strength and Conditioning Journal*, 32(3), 33–46. doi: 10.1519/ssc.0b013e3181df4521

This article, for the *Strength and Conditioning Journal*, was authored by Dr. Stuart McGill, a professor at the University of Waterloo in Ontario, Canada, and a world-renowned lecturer and expert in spine function, injury prevention, and rehabilitation.

The well-trained core is vital for optimum performance and injury prevention.

The core comprises the lumbar spine, muscles of the abdominal wall, back extensors, and quadratus lumborum. Included in the core are also multi-joint muscles, i.e., the latissimus dorsi and psoas which link the core to the pelvis, legs, shoulders, and arms. Because of the anatomical and biomechanical synergy with the pelvis, the gluteal muscles can additionally be considered essential components as primary power generators.

Core muscles, unlike limb muscles, co-contract, stiffening the torso in a way that allows all muscles to work together. Due to the importance of the core, McGill advocates training the core differently.

McGill states that in the personal training community, many advocate repeated spinal flexion (e.g., crunches or sit-ups) as a good method (often the solo method) to train the flexors (the rectus abdominis and the abdominal wall). However, these muscles are seldom used in this way.

More often they are used to brace while stopping motion. Consequently, they more frequently act as stabilizers, not flexors. McGill is adamant that repeated bending of the spinal discs is a potential injury concoction. McGill points out the misused practice of trainers having their clients pull in their abdominals to "activate their transverse abdominis," done in the name of enhancing stability. He explains that this does not target the major stabilizers of the spine because studies that measure stability show that the most important stabilizers are task specific.

For instance, sometimes the quadratus lumborum is most important, yet many coaches neglect this muscle. Second, drawing the abdominals inward actually reduces stability. Finally, evidence on transverse abdominis displays that activation disturbances may occur in some individuals with certain types of back disorders, but these same disturbances are not unique to transverse abdominis because they occur in many muscles.

The reality is clients are unable to activate this muscle in isolation (past extremely low levels of contraction) because it functions to activate with internal oblique muscles for athletic tasks.

Plenty of evidence demonstrates that the core makes the rest of the body perform better. For example, McGill's work on measuring the movements of strongman training established that the core-assisted hip function allows the strongmen to complete movements which they could not complete with hip strength alone.

Specifically, the quadratus lumborum aided in pelvis elevation to permit the swing leg to make a step. This suggests that a strong core allows strength to radiate out peripherally to more distant regions of the body.

The core usually functions to inhibit motion, not to initiate it. Optimal technique in most sporting and everyday living tasks demands that power be generated at the hips and transmitted through a stiffened core.

Instead of just performing traditional exercises like the squat, McGill suggests redirecting some of this activity with asymmetric carries such as the farmer's walk. McGill asserts that this builds the athleticism needed for many activities in a much more "spine friendly" way. The core is never a power generator. Rather, power is generated in the hips and transmitted through the stiffened core. Great athletes use the torso muscles as anti-motion controllers, rarely to generate motion (note, there are exceptions for throwers and the like, but the ones who create force pulses with larger deviations in spine posture are the ones who are usually injured first).

Takeaway Point

The core musculature must be very strong and capable of control to enhance training of other body regions and to facilitate optimal performance. Power training should be reserved for the hips, not the core. The bottom line is that many strongman events fit the bill!

Winwood, P. W., Cronin, J. B., Brown, S. R., and Keogh, J. W. L. (2015). A Biomechanical Analysis of the Strongman Log Lift and Comparison with Weightlifting's Clean and Jerk. *International Journal of Sports Science & Coaching*, 10(5), 869–886. doi: 10.1260/1747-9541.10.5.869

This study compared the biomechanical characteristics of the log lift with the clean and jerk. Six well-trained male strongman athletes performed log lifts and clean and jerks at 70% of their 1RM clean and jerk. The log lift demonstrated significantly greater trunk (↑24%) and hip (↑9%) range of motion compared to the clean and jerk. Notably greater peak bar velocities were achieved in the clean and jerk in the second pull (16%) and the jerk (↑14%). Interestingly, similarities existed in ground reaction force data between the lifts. Yet, mean and peak powers were significantly greater (↑40% to ↑64%) in propulsive phases of the clean and jerk.

Researchers concluded that the log lift may be an effective conditioning stimulus to teach rapid triple extension while generating similar vertical and anterior-propulsive forces as the clean and jerk with the same given load.

Takeaway Point

The log lift has a much simpler learning curve than the clean and jerk. So, unless someone is a competitive Olympic lifter, opt for the technically simpler movement that offers a similar training effect.

West, D. J., Cunningham, D. J., Finn, C. V., Scott, P. M., Crewther, B. T., Cook, C. J., and Kilduff, L. P. (2014). The Metabolic, Hormonal, Biochemical, and Neuromuscular Function Responses to a Backward Sled Drag Training Session. *Journal of Strength and Conditioning Research*, 28(1), 265–272. doi: 10.1519/jsc.0b013e3182948110

This study examined the metabolic, hormonal, biochemical, and neuromuscular function responses to a backward sled dragging session in strength-trained men. The study concluded that sled dragging provides an effective metabolic stimulus, with neuromuscular function (NMF) restored after three hours of recovery.

Maximal backward sled dragging provides a sufficient stimulus to place stress on multiple systems associated with athletic performance (e.g., strength endurance, metabolic, and hormonal), yet does not induce muscle damage and only acutely decreases NMF. With NMF restored after three hours, sled dragging offers athletes and strength coaches a training tool that requires limited recovery time and provides enough stress to promote favorable changes in baseline testosterone concentrations. Although there is potential for this training to induce some degree of muscle glycogen depletion, it is important to consider that as muscle damage was likely negated, there would be no hindrance to glycogen resynthesis.

The researchers' data supports the use of concentric-only training as a means to elicit favorable physiological responses in strength-trained athletes. This is huge because of the potential for traditional training methods to induce muscle damage and reduce NMF for approximately 48 hours. The recovery of NMF within three hours of a sled training session potentially allows athletes to execute additional training sessions. In addition, this type of exercise could be used as a means of active recovery.

Takeaway Point

Backward sled dragging is a low-risk, high-reward strength-training modality and can be huge for the battle-ridden injured traditional or tactical athlete.

Final Thoughts

Initially, strongman training outside of the sport of strongman was opposed by gung-ho Olympic lifting junky strength coaches who were set in their antiquated ways. Strongman training was also criticized by physically flaccid “lab coats” with no in-the-trenches experience who just wanted to take the company line.

Logically, strongman training makes sense, and its value is scientifically supported.

Interviews

While it’s essential to hear from the academics and experts in the labs and libraries, sometimes you want to hear firsthand from the athletes on the front lines in the battle for the acquisition of strength.

So, we sat down with a number of strength athletes and asked them about programs, personal experiences, and pearls of wisdom.

Take their advice as it serves you and your training.

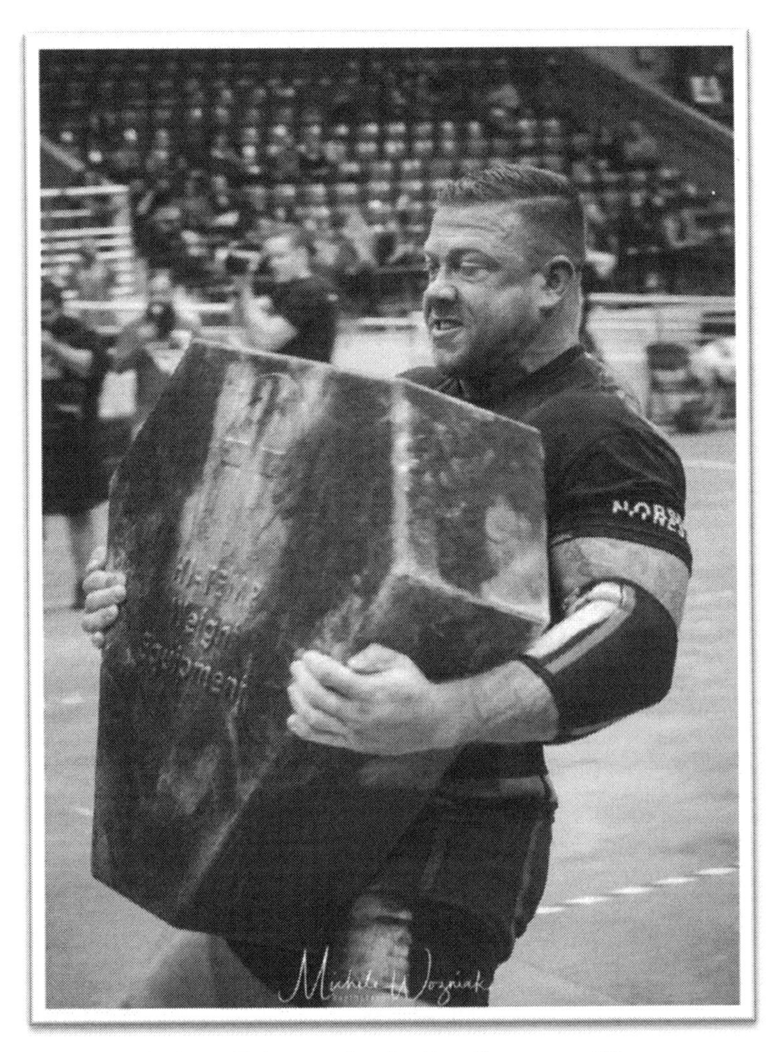

Anthony Fuhrman dominating the competition

Name: Anthony Fuhrman

Age: 31

Platoon Sergeant, US Army Warrior Fitness Team

2x 105kg WSM

1. How did you get started in the sport of strongman?

I started lifting with "bro" gym lifts. After I couldn't run anymore, I found alternate means to stay in shape and tried strongman training. I got in better shape in all metrics.

There was a tactical program for the 4th Infantry Division, and I was asked to try out stones. My first time trying atlas stones I loaded a 300+ pound stone and knew it was a match made in heaven. I have been training for five years now.

2. Who has inspired you in your strongman journey?

There are too many to list! Everyone in competitions has been able to provide something valuable.

3. How does your training split look in preparation for a contest?

Training is similar in-season and off-season; off-season usually has more hypertrophy.

4. Has strongman training helped you add muscle hypertrophy?

Absolutely! 100% it builds a physique—just look at the guys with massive backs all over the sport.

5. Has strongman training helped you gain strength in traditional lifts like the powerlifts?

Absolutely. I've done one powerlifting meet, and it was a month and a half after a strongman competition. I totaled 1,830 pounds at 242.

6. What advice do you have for someone training strongman at a commercial gym?

You have to get creative! My first two years as a professional, I had to train at a CrossFit gym. I didn't have equipment like a circus dumbbell, so I did a lot of single-arm barbell snatches. I didn't have stones to train with, so I'd stack 45s on a stand, pick them up, and walk with them.

This is a great option for object carries; it trains you to pull the weight into you.

7. How strong should someone be before entering a strongman contest?

Competing is worth it for anyone.

8. Is there a training program that has worked well for you for strongman preparation or a specific event?

Incorporating EMOM (Every Minute on the Minute) with strength training. For example, deadlifting one or two reps every minute on the minute at 80 percent for 10 straight minutes.

Strongman is about work capacity, not necessarily static strength.

I like to use some techniques from old-school John Meadows "Mountain Dog" Training, like "priming" before a major movement. I will do 20 to 30 hamstring curls before squats; it primes the movement.

Accessory moves are used with intensity to mimic strongman. Intense sets can get you ready for intense 60-second events in competition.

9. Do you feel strongman events could benefit tactical athletes' (police and military) strength and conditioning programs?

Yes. To be a tactical athlete is to train for strongman with modifications. There needs to be much more endurance, but it is the exact same movements. For example, carries should be done for 200 meters instead of 50 feet.

10. Any parting words of advice for our readers?

First off, reach out to somebody. Find someone; there is definitely at least one person in your area who can help you.

Second, use your imagination when training. Nothing works unless you try it!

"People like to be comfortable more than anything."

11. How can readers contact you?

IG @AnthonyFuhrmanStrong

12. Do you offer any online or coaching services?

Yes.

Name: Brittany Diamond

Age: 27

Pro Strongwoman, 3rd Strongest Woman in the World, Competitive Powerlifter

1. How did you get started strength training?

When I was in middle school, I would travel to the high school during the winter to run with the older, faster girls. I was obsessed with the idea of becoming faster and read all different magazines and books about strength training. I started squatting and lunging with dumbbells a few times a week after practice.

In high school, I worked in the weight room at my local YMCA, and I started incorporating upper body because I felt my arms were disproportionate compared to my lower body. I would do the basics—shoulder press, biceps curls, and push-ups. Tenth grade is when I touched a barbell for the first time after being introduced to the bench press from a gym teacher.

In college, I was a DI rower, but it's here that I fell in love with the process of strength training.

As rowers, we were tested on seal rows and front squats, and I can confidently say these two lifts gave me a solid foundation for strongman. It was in 2010 that I was introduced to programming for the first time and was fascinated by this idea that you could get better at basically everything by becoming stronger.

2. How did you get started in the sport of strongman?

The summer of 2013 I was home on break during my junior year of college. I worked part-time coaching high school girls at Grid Iron gym, a strength-training facility out of Woburn, MA. I was helping plan an event when I stumbled across an event called Boston's Strongest on Facebook; it was a local strongman show coming up at a nearby gym called Total Performance Sports. I vividly remember getting excited and thinking, "I love to lift and think I'm decently strong; this is for me!"

I signed up for women's novice and competed in the show two weeks later. I had never touched any of the implements, so I was just winging it. I watched videos online and read about various strongman techniques the week prior. To my surprise, I ended up placing first, and I was hooked.

During the competition, I felt a passion emerge that I hadn't felt in some time. I had LOVED track; rowing was a tough sport, but it wasn't a solo sport, and that is where I excelled.

Strongman lit a fire inside of me, and I knew I would take this sport as far as I could.

3. Who has inspired you in your strongman journey?

Eric Dawson, who is the owner of Titan Barbell, is my strongman dad. I met him at TPS at my first show, later finding out he was a pro strongman. He has a love for strongman, coaching, and all feats of strength. He ended up opening his own gym in June 2014—Titan Barbell right outside of Boston.

Titan Barbell was a facility run out of Eric's garage and my sanctuary. Every Saturday was "Strongman Saturday," and you could find me and several other dedicated athletes putting our bodies and minds to the test with various implements in Titan Barbell.

From the age of 22 to 25, I trained religiously at Titan Barbell and dedicated Saturdays to events.

It was at Titan, and under Eric's guidance, that I went from amateur to pro. There was one time I had to miss a Saturday for my brother's wedding, so Eric let me train on a Sunday.

He inspired me most by showing me the sacrifice and pain it would take to get to where I wanted to be athletically. Other people I had met in the industry dedicated their entire life to strongman.

While Eric certainly dedicated himself, he had a family, a business, and coached others, whom he also treated like family. He impacted me most by demonstrating how crazy strong one could be, but also how to treat others with respect and kindness no matter the circumstances.

4. How does your training split look in preparation for a contest?

The beauty of strongman is that every competition can vary greatly. Since a strongman athlete needs to be statically strong, be explosive, have endurance, and be technically sound, there are many moving parts. The first step when I am training for a specific contest is to identify my strengths and weaknesses in the events. I also map out what equipment I have available and when I can travel to get my hands on certain implements.

Generally, I will lift four times a week with a deadlift/squat day, two pressing days (one being heavier and event specific, and one concentrated more on technique/lighter weight), an event day where I simulate the contest, and two out of the four lifting days will involve some type of interval training. I like to pick an event to do my interval training with. Just to name a few examples: running with a sandbag or odd object, cleaning a log multiple times with no rest, sprinting with a sled. I'll program in the work times and rest times. Most strongman events are 60 seconds in duration, and no matter how strong you are, if you don't have the work capacity, you won't be successful in strongman. Occasionally, there's max time/max distance events, and the interval training will pay off dividends. I have excelled in moving events in strongman and know that my endurance background and "doing more cardio" than the average strongman athlete has paid off. I know that I typically program in more conditioning than other strongman coaches, but I make it as specific as possible.

As I've gone from novice to professional, I have stopped relying on implement training as much and concentrate more on static strength specifically focused around the big four (yes, there's four in strongman): squat, bench, deadlift, and overhead press. Since events are so heavy and can wreak havoc on your CNS and I have enough experience, I generally do not touch events until I am eight weeks out. I have always been a mover when it comes to strongman but have struggled with static events.

As I've gotten more experienced, I have also added in a fifth day of training where I focus primarily on movement patterns, mobility, and technical movements. This has helped me recover from injuries, avoid injuries that often happen with strongman training, and forced me to be more present with my body, which pays off during a competition.

When competing, I have always had a coach because it's important to have someone else's eye on you to see anything you may be missing and to get new ideas. Eric Dawson was my coach in the beginning, and he helped me earn my pro card with his constant attention to detail. I then coached myself for a while, only to realize how truly helpful and less stressful it was to have another opinion. I hired Josh Bryant, who had a very different training style than I was used to.

5. How does your training split look in the off-season?

In the off-season I incorporate much more volume than I would leading up to a contest, and it's an opportunity to troubleshoot. What I mean by troubleshoot is: identify my areas of weakness (being as specific as possible) and plan a course of action. For example, I've always struggled with the topmost portion (the lockout) of any overhead press; this comes down to popping my head through the keyhole and triceps strength. During the off-season, I'll be able to allot more time to hitting my triceps more frequently/multiple times a week.

A typical off-season training week will be five to six times of lifting, but the sessions are shorter since I don't have to warm up as much when I am not training implements/getting ready for an extremely heavy load. I am always working with submaximal weights and very rarely go above 85 percent on any lifts. I still train heavy, but you won't find me testing my 1rm. As I've gotten older especially, more volume works best for me. I will still touch events from time to time, but they are not as much of a priority as using the barbell, dumbbells, kettlebells, and machines.

Deadlifting off the floor is something I try to really focus on in the off-season because when you are in contest prep, you will certainly be deadlifting, but it's generally event specific. For example, an axle wagon wheel deadlift is a common strongman event. The wagon wheels make it so you are pulling approximately 16 to 18 inches raised. It's also important to note that as a strongman athlete, keeping a healthy lower back is a priority as it's generally the #1 injury a strongman athlete will see.

I like to combine strongman and bodybuilding together, and it's something I've been focusing on the last two years specifically working with Josh Bryant. Think about it: In bodybuilding-style training, you're focused on isolating each muscle, and the mind-muscle connection must be present. This works to your advantage because it gives you the opportunity to focus on specific areas.

6. Has strongman training helped you add muscle hypertrophy?

Absolutely. Lifting heavy and focusing on events that utilize every part of my muscle have helped me develop a strong, sturdy "powerhouse"-type physique. In strongman you use your back, legs, and grip for nearly everything and have to rely on full-body strength. You can do all the different variations of biceps exercises you can think of, but try lifting a stone three times your bodyweight for reps, and I guarantee you will feel muscles you can't hit from isolation exercises.

7. Has strongman training helped you gain strength in traditional lifts like the powerlifts?

Yes, going back to how nearly every event utilizes your full body, it absolutely transfers to the big three. There is always some sort of deadlift in a strongman contest, sometimes a squat, and while there isn't bench, overhead pressing will benefit your OHP and vice versa.

8. What advice do you have for someone training strongman at a commercial gym?
Take the time to map out a creative training plan. I had to train primarily in commercial gyms leading up to Strongest Woman in the World 2018 due to my travel schedule. Think of ways you can simulate the events. For example, walking with a trap bar can simulate frame/farmer's, bumper plates can simulate odd objects, a football bar can simulate a log. Although it's not ideal, strong is strong. Fat Gripz are an inexpensive tool you should have in your gym bag because incorporating more grip work will always help with strongman.

9. What gym lifts do you feel transfer best to static pressing events? Any general advice for athletes looking to increase static pressing strength?
Aside from static pressing itself, two important things are often overlooked: Increasing triceps strength and doing accessory work specific to moving heavy weight. While triceps pushdowns have their place, heavy, close-grip board presses are going to get you closer to your goal of building your press.

Keeping the shoulders healthy. This is often overlooked until it's too late. Taking care of shoulder mobility with things like YTWL and Cuban presses pays dividends in relation to not letting injury get in the way of your training.

10. What gym lifts do you feel transfer best to clean and jerk events? Any general advice for athletes looking to increase clean and jerk vent strength?
The clean and jerk, in my opinion, is the most technical event. Increasing your static press and push press will help your ability to move more weight, but it's equally as important to identify where your technical weakness is with this specific movement and find ways to mimic that part of the lift multiple times throughout the week. Submaximal weight for reps on reps helps your brain and body remember good movement patterns.

11. What gym lifts do you feel transfer best to loading events? Any general advice for athletes looking to increase loading event strength?
Front squats and Zercher squats have always been my favorite lifts when I don't have access to loading events themselves. They hit the upper back and fry your core more than any other lift.

Add in some three – to five-second pauses to toughen you up a bit, and you will be more prepared for a loading event once you get your hands on them.

12. What gym lifts do you feel transfer best to carrying events? Any general advice for athletes looking to increase carrying event strength?
The good news for practicing carrying events is that you don't need anything fancy. Simply walking around with a loaded SSB bar, heavy DBs in your hands, or carrying bumper plates will suffice, as long as you aim to move as quickly as possible with the weight. I see too many people always going heavy, and training for speed is how you get fast at moving events.

13. What gym lifts do you feel transfer best to holding events? Any general advice for athletes looking to increase holding event strength?
Dead hangs and what I've termed "Diamond Dead hangs" are some of my favorite ways to train holding events, and you can do them anywhere. To perform a diamond dead hang, you start in a regular dead hang

off of a neutral-grip pull-up bar, machine, or whatever you have. You hold your bodyweight as long as you can and then, starting with your nondominant hand, you hold yourself up with only that hand, then switch arms. Once you can get past 60 seconds all three ways, I recommend adding weight.

14. What gym lifts do you feel transfer best to deadlift events? Any general advice for athletes looking to increase deadlift event strength?

Deadlifting from a deficit and with an axle is a sure way not only to increase your 1rm in a barbell deadlift but also to prepare for strongman. In strongman you should always deadlift with the stiffest bar possible; adding in the axle adds in a great deal of difficulty, plus you will be using grip as well.

15. What gym lifts do you feel transfer best to throwing events? Any general advice for athletes looking to increase throwing event prowess?

Explosive warm-ups with medicine balls, such as the broad jump chest pass and overhead toss.

16. How strong should someone be before entering a strongman contest?

You should not set specific limitations on your strength before deciding to enter a contest. I feel you should have at least two years of general strength training under your belt, but it's better to enter a contest sooner rather than later so you can get the experience and then approach training knowing exactly what you need to hone in on.

17. Is there a training program that has worked well for you for strongman preparation or a specific event?

General linear progression and the cube method for strongman is how I started out. In the beginning, you don't need to worry about the perfect training plan; you just need to get stronger and get introduced to events.

18. Do you feel strongman events could benefit tactical athletes' (police and military) strength and conditioning programs?

100 percent, strongman will make you more efficient at moving heavy things faster, which is something police/military must be efficient in. For general strength and conditioning, strongman is built on a solid foundation of strength and conditioning, so the two go hand in hand.

19. How do you think strongman training can benefit tactical athletes?

You have to be well rounded on the battlefield, and being strong and efficient with moving things is a must.

20. How do you think strongman training can benefit other contact sports, for example, MMA, football, etc.?

Having experience with strongman can benefit you when you play contact sports because you'll have more power and knowledge than your opponent. With strongman, you have to have the ability to think fast in terms of deciding what the best way to do something is. Often, you may never get the chance to try an event until it's contest time. This can transfer to contact sports in the sense that it gives you an advantage over your opponents by being able to think plays through more efficiently.

20. Any parting words of advice for our readers?

You will NEVER feel strong or fast enough; it's the never-ending pursuit to strongman. The key is to be as prepared as you can be. DO NOT underestimate the power of a deload; you need adequate rest and recovery to give 100 percent.

21. How can readers contact you?

Instagram @B_Dimez or BDimezTraining.com

22. Do you offer any online or coaching services?

I specialize in guiding strongman competitors in season. I require at least 16 weeks of contest prep.

Name: Tom Sroka

Age: 33
American Open 105kg+ Champion 2013
Highland Games Pro
4th in the world in MAS Wrestling
442 c&j, 333 snatch

1. How did you get started strength training?

I was a shot-putter in college, and a three-time All-American in weight/hammer throw. I got involved in highland games and strongman after graduating. I was then recruited for Olympic lifting, and I competed in 2012 to 2016.

2. How did you get started in the sport of strongman?

I trained in a garage for a long time and was constantly making equipment, improvising, and testing random training methods to see what worked.

3. What advice do you have for someone training strongman at a commercial gym?

Network, especially on social media; there are great people on it. If you don't know something, ask; you will be surprised who may respond and give you helpful information.

Always be curious: Go on elitefts, Instagram, etc., to find people who can help you. They are out there. Always be learning.

4. How do you think strongman training can benefit tactical athletes?

When it comes to training anybody, no matter what, the big thing is people need to know how to use their body in space and know what their body is capable of. We do a lot of GPP, including carries, sandbags, diverse movements, calisthenics. Even though it seems boring, the expansion you can get on those is enormous and endless, versus if you start with bands and chains, you don't have many places to go and can't do an air squat.

EVERYBODY goes through the same basics, and then we'll see what the next step is for that person.

Strongman/functional strength training is perfect for anyone; it just requires modifications and specifications for the goal.

5. Any parting words of advice for our readers?

Start small, build big!

6. How can readers contact you?

Tom@thestrengthagenda.com
Strength_coach_sroka
@thestrengthagenda

7. Do you offer any online or coaching services?

Yes!

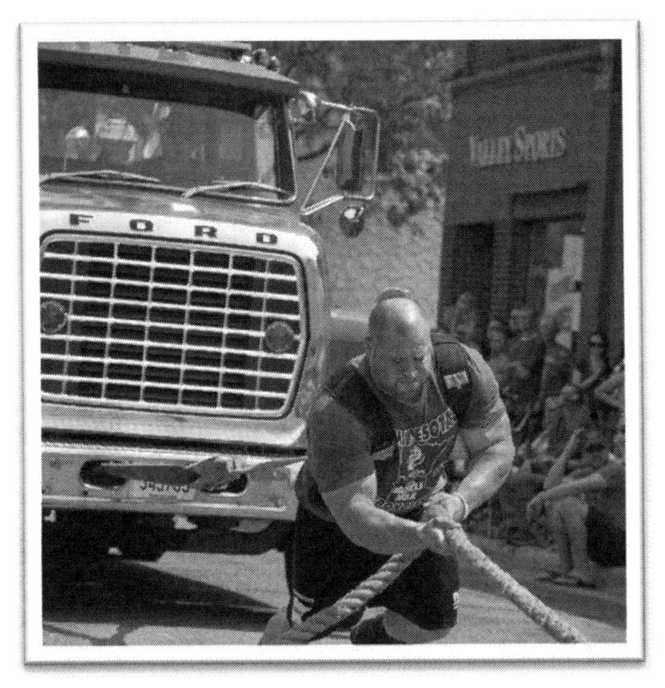

Joel Dirks Truck Pull

Name: Joel Dirks

Pro Strongman
Age: 36

1. How did you get started strength training?

Toward the end of 9th grade. In 10th grade I got more serious for football.

2. How did you get started in the sport of strongman?

After I was done in college football and track, I still had the drive to compete. I saw a local competition with a guy pulling a truck and knew it was the perfect fit. I messaged Dave Ostlund, who had just placed third at

World's Strongest Man in 2008, and started training with him. My first competition was in 2009 and first pro show in 2011.

3. Who has inspired you in your strongman journey?

My inspiration was to win the Arnold Amateur; it had started at the same time I started competing.

4. How does your training split look in preparation for a contest?

Usually always a press day and deadlift day. A typical week looks like:

Monday: Pressing (axle or log) and accessories (This is event specific for the competition; I will train reps or maxes depending on what the event is.)

Tuesday: Front squats and leg accessories

Wednesday: Off from lifting; I do tons of mobility, fascia release, and other methods as needed

Thursday: Deadlifts and back accessories

Friday: Same as Wednesday

Saturday: Events—depends on the upcoming competition

Sunday: Off

5. How does your training split look in the off-season?

Monday: Pressing

Tuesday: Squats

Wednesday: Off

Thursday: Incline and Upper Body

Friday: Deadlift

Weekend: Off

6. Has strongman training helped you add muscle hypertrophy?

Yes, 100 percent.

7. Has strongman training helped you gain strength in traditional lifts like the powerlifts?

Yes, 100 percent.

8. What advice do you have for someone training strongman at a commercial gym?

Get creative: Turn a Hex bar into a car deadlift; press in different ways, such as a circus DB with fat grips.

Build your foundation in static strength.

9. What gym lifts do you feel transfer best to static pressing events? Any general advice for athletes looking to increase static pressing strength?

Standing strict press out of the rack—barbell bench does not have a huge carryover, so focus on strict pressing.

10. What gym lifts do you feel transfer best to clean and jerk events? Any general advice for athletes looking to increase clean and jerk event strength?

Cleans, especially on the axle work, squats, and heavy upright rows

11. What gym lifts do you feel transfer best to loading events? Any general advice for athletes looking to increase loading event strength?

Pick up any odd objects you have access to; that always helps with loads.

12. What gym lifts do you feel transfer best to holding events? Any general advice for athletes looking to increase holding event strength?

Farmer hold for time. Load up the heaviest weight you can use and hold for 45 seconds.

13. What gym lifts do you feel transfer best to deadlift events? Any general advice for athletes looking to increase deadlift event strength?

Deadlifts!

14. How strong should someone be before entering a strongman contest?

What's important is to compete! Do the events regardless of how you will do. You will meet people with equipment, who live close, who will help your training, etc., and you'll get experience.

15. Do you feel strongman events could benefit tactical athletes' (police and military) strength and conditioning programs?

Yes! Strongman training—regardless of what you're trying to do—will improve your mobility while you're under a load.

Strongman training is also beneficial to powerlifting as well because it makes you well rounded; you have to be good at everything instead of just technically sound at three lifts.

16. Any parting words of advice for our readers?

Strongman is a great way to spice up your training. It's much more fun than conventional lifts and provides a challenge unlike any other modality.

Competitions give you a purpose, leading you to better-focused training blocks.

17. How can readers contact you?

IG: @JoelDirks

IG: @American.Strength1776

18. Do you offer any online or coaching services?

Yes.

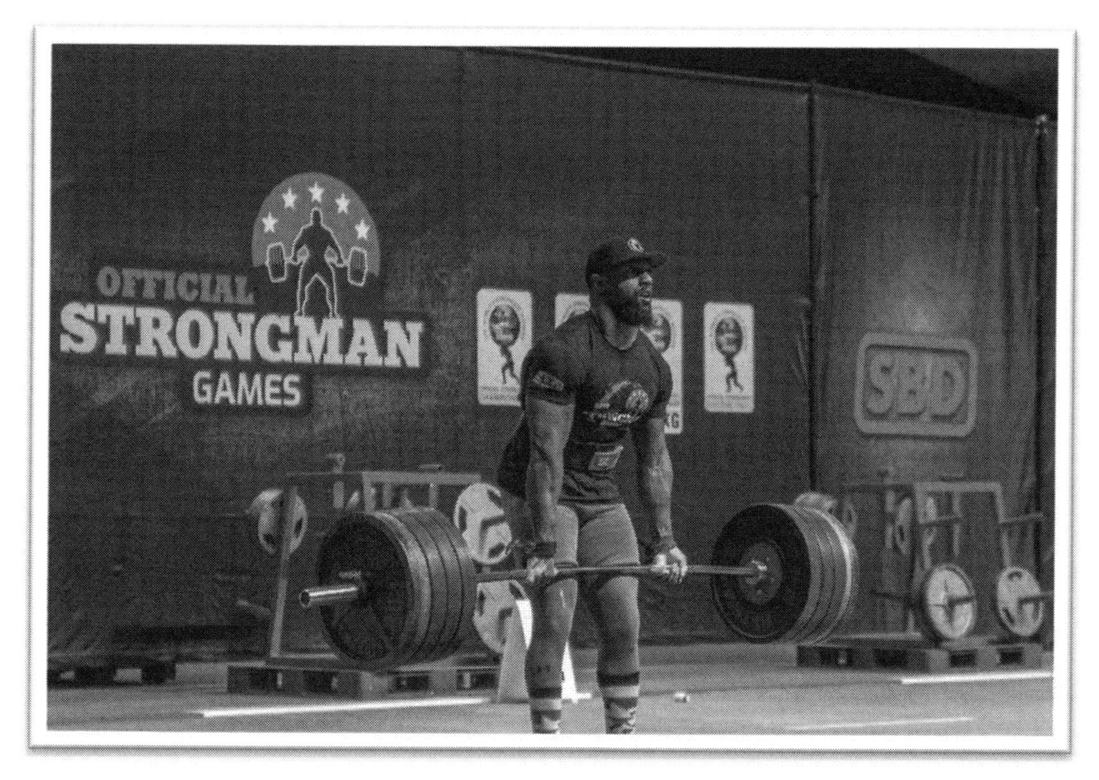

Mark Jones Deadlift

Name: Mark Jones

World's Strongest Man under 90kg, Competitive Bodybuilder

Strongman is a community—everyone wants to see everyone succeed and lift heavy shit.

Competitors are high-fiving in the back, using each other's massagers and rollers—it's a real family. It takes a special type of athlete to support your fellow competitor.

1. How did you get started strength training?

I have always had an athletic background. I ran track in high school and played college football at Youngstown. I got a job at campus rec and started to lift more seriously.

2. How did you get started in the sport of strongman?

I was invited to a gym that had metabolic training and bootcamp workouts that included odd objects like farmer's carries and kegs. Lifting odd objects became an obsession, which led me to a desire to compete.

3. Who has inspired you in your strongman journey?

Mark and Sean Shoemaker

4. How does your training change for bodybuilding and strongman?

Yes, I won a bodybuilding show one week before winning a strongman competition. My workouts never changed, just the diet. It was all functional training. I had so much girth and size because I wasn't doing the traditional bodybuilding hypertrophy stuff.

5. Has strongman training helped you gain strength in traditional lifts like the powerlifts?

Yes. I competed in the XPC Deadlift Salute at the Arnold and pulled 765 as a lightweight. My previous highest deadlift attempt before this was a failed 725.

6. What advice do you have for someone training strongman at a commercial gym?

Train for time, conditioning style, instead of reps. Do five rounds of 30 seconds on an accessory instead of just straight repetitions.

Strongman came from limited equipment, so you have to maximize yourself with anything you have. Try to do things in an unorthodox way; use fat grips, towels for pull-ups, anything you can.

7. Any parting words of advice for our readers?

Athletes come in all shapes and sizes. Not everyone is built the same; be comfortable in the abilities you have and keep building from there! Work on your weaknesses—that's what will make you better.

You have to be ready mentally for anything. Even if it means going to a dark place and risking injury or blacking out, you have to be ready.

8. How can readers contact you?

IG @Jones_BSSStrong

9. Do you offer any online or coaching services?

No.

Made in the USA
Middletown, DE
27 May 2024